PocketRadiologist™
Vascular
Top 100 Diagnoses

PocketRadiologist™
Vascular
Top 100 Diagnoses

William G Bradley Jr MD PhD
Professor and Chairman, Department of Radiology
University of California San Diego
San Diego, California

William J Zwiebel MD
Professor of Radiology, University of Utah School of Medicine
Staff Radiologist, VA Salt Lake City Health Care System
Salt Lake City, Utah

Anne Roberts MD
Professor of Radiology
University of California San Diego
LaJolla, California

Anne G Osborn MD
University Distinguished Professor of Radiology
William H and Patricia W Child Presidential Endowed Chairholder
University of Utah School of Medicine
Salt Lake City, Utah

Amersham Health Visiting Professor in Diagnostic Imaging
Armed Force Insititue of Pathology
Washington, DC

H Ric Harnsberger MD
Professor of Radiology
R C Willey Chair in Neuroradiology
University of Utah School of Medicine
Salt Lake City, Utah

Lawrence N Tanenbaum MD
Section Chief MRI, CT and Neuroradiology
Edison Imaging / New Jersey Neuroscience Institute
Edison, New Jersey

PocketRadiologist™
Vascular
Top 100 Diagnoses

Additional contributions by:

> Michele Brown MD
> Eric Chen MD
> Lane F Donnelly MD
> Thomas M Grist MD
> Gabriella Iussich MD
> Barry Katzen MD
> John Kaufman MD
> Tom Kinney MD
> Kevin R Moore MD
> Karen L Salzman MD
> Richard H Wiggins III MD

With 200 drawings and radiographic images

Drawings:	Lane R Bennion MS
	Richard Coombs MS
	James A Cooper MD
	Jill Rhead MA
	Walter Stuart MFA
Image Editing:	Ming Q Huang MD
	Danielle Morris
	Melissa Petersen
Medical Text Editing:	Richard H Wiggins III MD

AMIRSYS™

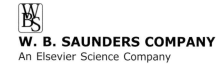

W. B. SAUNDERS COMPANY
An Elsevier Science Company

AMIRSYS™

A medical reference publishing company

First Edition

First Printing: November 2002

Composition by Amirsys Inc, Salt Lake City, Utah

Printed by K/P Corporation, Salt Lake City, Utah

ISBN: 0-7216-0037-9

Preface

The **PocketRadiologist™** series is an innovative, quick reference designed to deliver succinct, up-to-date information to practicing professionals "at the point of service." As close as your pocket, each title in the series is written by world-renowned authors. These experts have designated the "top 100" diagnoses or interventional procedures in every major body area, bulleted the most essential facts, and offered high-resolution imaging to illustrate each topic. Selected references are included for further review. Full color anatomic-pathologic computer graphics model many of the actual diseases.

Each **PocketRadiologist™** title follows an identical format. The same information is in the same place - every time - and takes you quickly from key facts to imaging findings, differential diagnosis, pathology, pathophysiology, and relevant clinical information. The interventional modules give you the essentials and "how-tos" of important procedures, including pre- and post-procedure checklists, common problems and complications.

PocketRadiologist™ titles are available in both print and hand-held PDA formats. Currently available modules feature Brain, Head and Neck, Orthopedic (Musculoskeletal) Imaging, Pediatrics, Spine, Chest, Cardiac, Vascular, Abdominal Imaging and Interventional Radiology. 2003 topics will include Obstetrics, Gynecologic Imaging, Breast, and much, much more. Enjoy!

Anne G Osborn MD
Editor-in-Chief, Amirsys Inc

H Ric Harnsberger MD
Chairman and CEO, Amirsys Inc

Notice and Disclaimer

The information in this product ("Product") is provided as a reference for use by licensed medical professionals and no others. It does not and should not be construed as any form of medical diagnosis or professional medical advice on any matter. Receipt or use of this Product, in whole or in part, does not constitute or create a doctor-patient, therapist-patient, or other healthcare professional relationship between Amirsys Inc. ("Amirsys") and any recipient. This Product may not reflect the most current medical developments, and Amirsys makes no claims, promises, or guarantees about accuracy, completeness, or adequacy of the information contained in or linked to the Product. The Product is not a substitute for or replacement of professional medical judgment. Amirsys and its affiliates, authors, contributors, partners, and sponsors disclaim all liability or responsibility for any injury and/or damage to persons or property in respect to actions taken or not taken based on any and all Product information.

In the cases where drugs or other chemicals are prescribed, readers are advised to check the Product information currently provided by the manufacturer of each drug to be administered to verify the recommended dose, the method and duration of administration, and contraindications. It is the responsibility of the treating physician relying on experience and knowledge of the patient to determine dosages and the best treatment for the patient.

To the maximum extent permitted by applicable law, Amirsys provides the Product AS IS AND WITH ALL FAULTS, AND HEREBY DISCLAIMS ALL WARRANTIES AND CONDITIONS, WHETHER EXPRESS, IMPLIED OR STATUTORY, INCLUDING BUT NOT LIMITED TO, ANY (IF ANY) IMPLIED WARRANTIES OR CONDITIONS OF MERCHANTABILITY, OF FITNESS FOR A PARTICULAR PURPOSE, OF LACK OF VIRUSES, OR ACCURACY OR COMPLETENESS OF RESPONSES, OR RESULTS, AND OF LACK OF NEGLIGENCE OR LACK OF WORKMANLIKE EFFORT. ALSO, THERE IS NO WARRANTY OR CONDITION OF TITLE, QUIET ENJOYMENT, QUIET POSSESSION, CORRESPONDENCE TO DESCRIPTION OR NON-INFRINGEMENT, WITH REGARD TO THE PRODUCT. THE ENTIRE RISK AS TO THE QUALITY OF OR ARISING OUT OF USE OR PERFORMANCE OF THE PRODUCT REMAINS WITH THE READER.

Amirsys disclaims all warranties of any kind if the Product was customized, repackaged or altered in any way by any third party.

PocketRadiologist™
Vascular
Top 100 Diagnoses

The diagnoses in this book are divided into 7 sections in the following order:

Brain
Head & Neck
Spine
Thorax
Abdominal
Renal
Upper/Lower Extremity

Table of Contents

Brain

Head & Neck

Table of Contents

Spine

Thorax

Abdominal

Renal

Upper/Lower Extremity

Table of Contents

PocketRadiologist™
Vascular
Top 100 Diagnoses

BRAIN

Persistent Trigeminal Artery

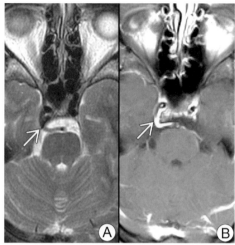

Persistent trigeminal artery (PTA). Axial T2WI (A) and contrast enhanced T1WI (B) show a persistent trigeminal artery (arrows). (Courtesy Anne G Osborn MD)

Key Facts
- Definition: Persistent (embryonic) carotid basilar anastomosis (PCBA) between cavernous ICA and basilar artery (BA)
- Classic imaging appearance
  - Vascular channel from cavernous ICA courses posteriorly, then medially to join distal BA
  - Sagittal MR shows "trident sign"
- PTA = most common PCBA
  - Present in 0.1-0.2% of cerebral angiograms
- 25% prevalence of other vascular anomalies (e.g., aneurysm)
- Less common carotid-basilar communications
  - Persistent hypoglossal artery
  - Persistent otic artery
  - Proatlantal intersegmental artery

Imaging Findings
<u>General Features</u>
- Best imaging clue: Anomalous vessel bridges anterior (ICA) and posterior (BA) circulations **below** level of PCoA (circle of Willis)

<u>CT Findings</u>
- CECT: Large caliber vessel courses between basilar artery and ICA
- CTA delineates presence and course of vascular anomaly, associated abnormalities (e.g., saccular aneurysm)

<u>MR Findings</u>
- Prominent flow void bridging anterior and posterior circulation
  - Sagittal T1WI: Looks like "Neptune's trident"
  - Axial T1-, T2WI: Prominent but anomalous vessel passes posteriorly from ICA (either around or directly through dorsum sellae) to BA
- MRA readily depicts anatomical variant; careful (right-left) segmentation of MRA data advised to avoid misinterpretation

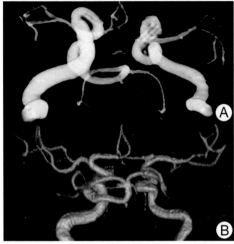

Persistent trigeminal artery. Inferior (A) and posterior (B) volume rendered MRA views demonstrate anomalous communication between ICA and hypoplastic basilar artery.

Angiography Findings
- Two types
  - Saltzman type I
    - PTA supplies entire distal vertebrobasilar system
    - BA below anastomosis usually hypoplastic
    - PCoAs usually absent
  - Saltzman type II
    - PTA fills superior cerebellar arteries
    - Posterior cerebral arteries supplied via patent PCoAs
- Other vascular anomalies in 25% of cases
  - Aneurysms in 10-15% of cases

Imaging Recommendations
- May be incidental finding on MR or CT
- Confirm with MRA or CTA
- Look for other vascular lesions

Differential Diagnosis: Persistent Carotid-Vertebrobasilar Anastomoses (CVBAs)

Persistent Hypoglossal Artery
- Second most common carotid vertebrobasillar anastomoses (CVBA)
  - Found in 0.03-0.26% of angiograms
  - Connects cervical ICA (approximately C1-2 level) with BA
  - Courses through enlarged hypoglossal canal, not foramen magnum
  - Partly parallels CN XII

Persistent Otic Artery (POA)
- Very rare
- Courses from petrous ICA through internal acoustic meatus to caudal BA
- Vertebral arteries may be absent or hypoplastic, therefore PSA may be dominant or only supply to basilar artery
- Rarely identified at angiography

Persistent Trigeminal Artery

Proatlantal Intersegmental Artery (PIA)
- Most caudal of PCBAs
- Originates from cervical ICA (approximately C2-3 level) or (less commonly) from ECA
- Communicates with **vertebral artery** coursing between the arch of C1 and occiput
- Vertebral arteries may be absent or hypoplastic, therefore PIA may be dominant or only supply to basilar artery

Pathology
General
- General Path Comments
  - Increased incidence of intracranial aneurysms and vascular malformations
- Embryology
  - Several transient segmental connections between primitive carotid, hindbrain circulations appear in early fetal development
  - Connections are named according to the cranial nerves they parallel
  - Embryonic trigeminal artery supplies basilar artery before definitive PCoA and vertebral arteries develop
  - Embryonic trigeminal artery usually regresses as definitive circulation develops
  - Failure to regress results in PTA
- Anatomy
  - PTA arises from cavernous ICA near posterior genus
  - Runs posterolaterally along trigeminal nerve (41%) or directly through dorsum sellae (59%)
  - Usually associated with small PCoA, vertebral arteries, proximally hypoplastic BA

Clinical Issues
Presentation
- Most common presentation: Incidental finding at imaging (anomalous vessel noted on MR/CT/DSA)
- May cause intracranial hemorrhage if other associated vascular anomaly is present
Treatment
- No treatment for PTA itself is required

Selected References
1. Suttner et al: Persistent trigeminal artery: A unique anatomic specimen – analysis and therpeutic implications. Neurosurg 47(2): 428-33, 2000
2. Silbergleit et al: Persistent trigeminal artery detected with standard MRI. JCAT 17: 22-25, 1993
3. Oshiro et al: Branches of the persistent primitive trigeminal artery: An autopsy case. Neurosurg 32: 144-8, 1993

Sturge-Weber Syndrome

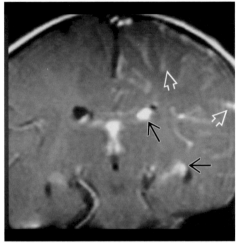

Contrast-enhanced T1W coronal image demonstrates leptomeningeal enhancement (open arrows) and enlarged, enhancing choroid plexi (black arrows).

Key Facts
- Synonym: SWS, encephalotrigeminal angiomatosis
- Definition: "Port wine stain" facial nevus
- Usually a sporadic congenital (but not inherited) malformation
- Fetal cortical veins fail to develop normally
- Imaging sequelae caused by **chronic venous ischemia**

Imaging Findings
General Features
- Best diagnostic sign = cortical Ca++/atrophy + enlarged choroid plexus
- Findings relate to sequelae of progressive venous occlusion
CT Findings
- NECT
  - o Gyral/subcortical white matter Ca++
    - Ca++ **not** in leptomeningeal angioma
    - Progressive, generally posterior to anterior (2-20y)
  - o Late
    - Atrophy
    - Hyperpneumatization of paranasal sinuses
    - Thick diploe
- CECT
  - o Serpentine leptomeningeal enhancement
  - o Ipsilateral choroid plexus enlargement almost universal
MR Findings
- Early: "Accelerated" myelin maturation 2° to transient hyp**er**perfusion
  - o Pial angioma, subarachnoid space vessels/trabeculae enhance
- Late: "Burnt-out" ⇒ ↓ pial enhancement, ↑ cortical/subcortical Ca++; atrophy, white matter gliosis (↑ signal T2)
Other Modality Findings
- DSA: Pial blush, paucity of normal cortical veins
- MRV

Sturge-Weber Syndrome

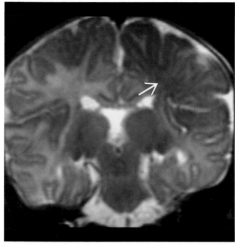

T2* weighted coronal demonstrates hypointense white matter (arrow) due to slow venous drainage and increased extraction of oxygen, i.e., increased deoxyhemoglobin.

- o Lack superficial cortical veins
- o ↓ Flow transverse sinuses/jugular veins
- o ↑↑ Prominence deep collateral (medullary/subependymal) veins
- o Progressive sinovenous occlusion
- PET: Progressive hypoperfusion/glucose hypometabolism
- MRS: ↓ NAA in affected areas
- SPECT: Transient hyperperfusion (early)
- Orbital enhancement > 50%

Imaging Recommendations (N.I.H.)
- MR with contrast (assess extent, uni-/bilaterality, orbital involvement)

Differential Diagnosis
Other Vascular Phakomatoses (Neurocutaneous Syndromes)
- Wyburn-Mason syndrome
  - o Facial vascular nevus
  - o Visual pathway and/or brain AVM
- Klippel-Trenaunay-Weber syndrome
  - o Osseous/soft-tissue hypertrophy, extremity vascular malformations
  - o May be combined with some features of SWS
- Meningioangiomatosis
  - o Ca++ common; variable leptomeningeal enhancement
  - o May invade brain through Virchow Robin space (VRSs)
  - o Atrophy usually absent

Celiac Disease
- Bilateral occipital Ca++
- Predominantly Mediterranean (Italian) ancestry
- No angiomatous involvement brain/face

Sturge-Weber Syndrome

Pathology

General

- General Path Comments
  - Cutaneous nevus flammeus CN V_1
  - +/- Visceral angiomatosis
- Genetics
  - Usually sporadic with no known inheritance
  - Very rare: Familial or with other vascular phakomatosis
- Embryology
  - Embryonic cortical veins fail to coalesce and develop
  - Persistence of primordial vessels
    - Occurs at 4-8 week stage
    - Visual cortex adjacent to optic vesicle and upper fetal face
- Etiology-Pathogenesis-Pathophysiology
  - Arrested development fetal vasculature $\Rightarrow$ deep venous occlusion, venous stasis $\Rightarrow$ anoxia cortex
- Epidemiology
  - Rare: 1:50,000

Gross Pathologic or Surgical Features

- Meningeal hypervascularity/angiomatosis
- Subjacent cortical/subcortical Ca++

Microscopic Features

- Pial angioma = multiple thin-walled vessels in enlarged sulci
- Cortical atrophy, Ca++

Clinical Issues

Presentation

- CN V_1 facial nevus flammeus ("port wine stain") 98%
- Pial angiomatosis unilateral 80%, bilateral 20%
  - Seizures 90%; hemiparesis 30–66%
  - Stroke-like episodes; neurological deficit 65%
- Eye findings esp. with upper and lower lid nevus flammeus
  - Choroidal angioma 70% $\Rightarrow$ $\uparrow$ intraocular pressure/congenital glaucoma $\Rightarrow$ buphthalmos
- Retinal telangiectatic vessels; scleral angioma; iris heterochromia
- Seizures (Sz) develop in first year of life
  - Infantile spasms $\Rightarrow$ tonic/clonic, myoclonic
  - If Sz $\Rightarrow$ developmental delay 43%, emotional/behavioral problems 85%, special education 70%, employability 46%
- Progressive hemiparesis 30%, homonymous hemianopsia 2%

Natural History

- Progressive Sz, neurological deficit, atrophy

Treatment & Prognosis

- $\uparrow$ Extent of lobar involvement, white matter alterations, and degree of atrophy $\Rightarrow$ $\uparrow$ likelihood Sz (also developmental delay)

Selected References

1. Maria BL et al: Central nervous system structure and function in Sturge-Weber syndrome: Evidence of neurologic and radiologic progression. J Child Neurol 13: 606-18, 1998
2. Sujansky E et al: Outcome of Sturge-Weber syndrome in 52 adults. Am J Med Genet 22; 57: 35-45, 1995
3. Braffman B et al: The Phakomatoses: Part II. Neuroimaging Clinics of North America 4: 325-48, 1994

Von Hippel-Lindau Disease

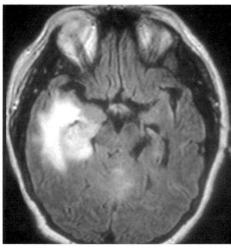

Large right temporal lobe mass with surrounding edema on unenhanced FLAIR proven to be hemangioblastoma in a 36-year-old woman with VHL with previous resections of cerebellar hemangioblastomas.

Key Facts
- Synonym: VHL
- Autosomal dominant hereditary tumor syndrome with high penetrance, variable expression
  - Affects six different organ systems, including eye and CNS
  - Involved tissues often have multiple lesions
  - Lesions = benign cysts, vascular tumors, carcinomas
- Phenotypes based on absence or presence of pheochromocytoma
  - Type 1 = without pheochromocytoma
  - Type 2A = with both pheochromocytoma and renal cell carcinoma
  - Type 3A = with pheochromocytoma, without renal cell carcinoma

Imaging Findings
General Features
- Varies with organ, lesion type
- Best diagnostic sign = 2 CNS hemangioblastomas or 1 + retinal hemorrhage

CT Findings
- NECT
  - 2/3 well-delineated cerebellar cyst + nodule, 1/3 solid
  - +/- Obstructive hydrocephalus
- CECT
  - Intense enhancement of solid nodule

MR Findings
- Contrast-enhancing nodule + cyst or syrinx (cord)
- May detect tiny enhancing nodules

Other Modality Findings
- DSA shows intensely vascular mass, prolonged stain

Imaging Recommendations (N.I.H.)
- Contrast-enhanced MR of brain/spinal cord from age 11y, every 2 years
- U/S of abdomen from 11y, yearly

Von Hippel-Lindau Disease

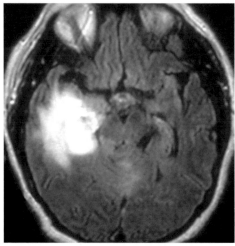

Same case as previous figure. Enhanced FLAIR image shows enhancing mass.

- Abdominal CT from 20y, yearly or every other year
- MRI of temporal bone if hearing loss, tinnitus/vertigo looking for endolymphatic sac tumor

Differential Diagnosis

Pilocytic Astrocytoma (Cerebellum)
- Different age (usually younger)

Metastasis
- Usually solid, not cyst + nodule
- Some tumors (e.g., renal clear cell carcinoma) can resemble hemangioblastoma histopathologically

Pathology

General
- General Path Comments
  - VHL characterized by development of
    - Capillary hemangioblastomas of the CNS and retina
    - Cysts, renal cell carcinoma
    - Pheochromocytoma
    - Pancreatic cysts, islet cell tumors
    - Inner ear (endolymphatic sac) tumors
    - Epididymal cysts, cystadenomas
- Genetics
  - Autosomal dominant inheritance
  - Germline mutations of VHL tumor suppressor gene
    - Chromosome 3p25-26
    - Involved in cell cycle regulation, angiogenesis
    - Different mutations scattered throughout gene
    - Disease features vary depending on specific VHL mutations
    - Inactivating mutations (nonsense mutations/deletions) predispose to VHL type 1
    - Missense mutations predispose to VHL types 2A, 2B

Von Hippel-Lindau Disease

- Etiology-Pathogenesis-Pathophysiology
  - Both alleles of tumor suppressor gene inactivated
  - Suppressor gene product = VHL protein
  - Mechanism by which neoplasia is induced unclear
- Epidemiology
  - 1 in 35-50,000 (no racial, gender predilection)
  - 25% of capillary hemangioblastomas associated with VHL

Gross Pathologic or Surgical Features
- Well-circumscribed, very vascular, reddish nodule
- 75% at least partially cystic, contain amber-colored fluid

Microscopic Features
- Two components
  - Rich capillary network
  - Large, vacuolated stromal cells with clear cytoplasm
- Immunohistochemistry = for cytokeratins, Lu-5

Staging or Grading Criteria
- Capillary hemangioblastoma = WHO grade I

Clinical Issues
Presentation
- Clinically heterogeneous; phenotypic penetrance = 97% at 65y
- Diagnosis of VHL = capillary hemangioblastoma in CNS/retina **and** one of typical VHL-associated tumors **or** previous family history
- Hemangioblastomas usually occur in adults
  - Retinal
    - Mean age = 25y
    - Visual symptoms (retinal detachment, vitreous hemorrhage)
  - Cerebellar
    - Mean age = 30y
    - Headache (obstructive hydrocephalus)
  - Spinal cord
    - Progressive myelopathy (tumor + syrinx)
- VHL-associated tumors
  - Pheochromocytoma (30y)
  - Renal carcinoma (33y)
  - Endolymphatic duct tumor

Natural History
- Renal carcinoma proximal cause of death in 15%-50%

Treatment & Prognosis
- Ophthalmoscopy yearly from infancy
- Physical/neurological examination, from 2y, yearly
- Surgical resection of symptomatic cerebellar/spinal hemangioblastoma
- Stereotactic radiosurgery may control smaller lesions
- Laser treatment of retinal angiomata

Selected References
1. Bohling T et al: Von Hippel-Lindau disease and capillary hemangioblastoma. In Kleihues P, Cavanee WK (eds): Tumours of the central nervous system, 223-6, IARC Press, 2000
2. Hes FJ et al: Von Hippel-Lindau disease: strategies in early detection (renal-, adrenal- pancreatic masses). Eur Radiol 9: 598-610, 1999
3. Neumann HPH et al: Von Hippel-Lindau syndrome. Brain Pathol 5: 181-93, 1995

Vein of Galen Malformation

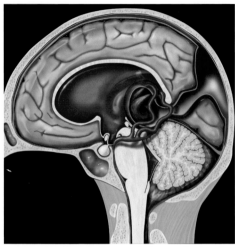

Illustration showing AVM with central venous drainage and enlarged vein of Galen, compressing aquaduct, leading to hydrocephalus.

Key Facts
- Synonym: Vein of Galen "aneurysm" (misnomer)
- Definition: Intracranial arteriovenous malformation involving aneurysmal dilatation of the vein of Galen
- Most common extracardiac cause of high-output congestive heart failure in neonatal period
- Classic plain film appearance: Global cardiomegaly, pulmonary vascular congestion, wide upper mediastinum
- Category: Acyanotic, cardiomegaly, increased pulmonary vascularity
- Hemodynamics
    o Large extracardiac left to right shunt
    o Volume overload of all cardiac chambers and great vessels

Imaging Findings
General Features
- Best imaging clue: Generalized dilatation of head and neck vessels
Chest Radiography
- Global cardiomegaly
- Increased pulmonary vascularity +/- pulmonary edema
- Large aortic knob, pulmonary artery segment
- Wide upper mediastinum due to dilatation of carotids and jugulars
Echocardiography
- Global cardiac chamber enlargement
- No structural cardiac abnormalities
- Dilated ascending aorta and its branches (carotid and vertebral arteries)
- Mild coarctation of aortic isthmus due to fetal flow dynamics (most of left ventricular output goes to cranial fistula)
- Dilated central veins with abnormally pulsatile flow signal
- Retrograde diastolic flow in descending aorta due to steal phenomenon

Vein of Galen Malformation

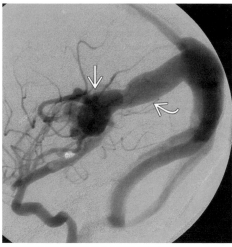

Left carotid angiogram lateral view, in a 3-year-old with a vein of Galen malformation (arrow). Note persistent falcine sinus (curved arrow), absent straight sinus.

Cranial Doppler Ultrasonography
- Large cystic structure in midline with turbulent pulsatile (arterialized) flow, draining into dilated straight sinus and torcula Herophili
- Feeding arteries and nidus may be identified (posterior choroidal, thalamoperforating, lenticulostriate and pericallosal arteries)
- Associated hydrocephalus, due to aqueductal compression
- Intracranial hemorrhage, ischemic lesions

CT Findings
- NECT: Dilated vein of Galen slightly hyperdense to brain parenchyma
  - +/- Hydrocephalus
  - +/- Intraventricular hemorrhage
  - Periventricular hypodensity ~ leukomalacia
- CECT: Strong enhancement of malformation including feeding arteries

MR Findings
- T1WI: Shows anatomy of malformation, associated findings (hydrocephalus, hemorrhage)
- T2WI: May show ischemic white matter disease due to arterial steal
- MRA, MRV: Improves delineation of feeding arteries, nidu, draining veins

Angiography
- Only required for attempt at staged embolization
- Selective carotid and vertebral artery injections
- Superselective injections prior to initial embolization of feeders
- Retrograde venous catheterization for deposition of coils in vein of Galen
- Multiple repeat treatments are often necessary

Imaging Recommendations
- Diagnosis often suspected with echocardiography
- Primary diagnosis confirmed with cranial Doppler ultrasound
- MRI/MRA for complete mapping of the lesion
- Angiography only for embolization treatment

Vein of Galen Malformation

Differential Diagnosis

Other Systemic Arteriovenous Malformations
- Single or multiple liver hemangiomas/hemangioendotheliomas
  - May require embolization or surgical ligation of hepatic artery
- Extremity or soft-tissue arteriovenous malformations/fistulae
  - Klippel-Trenaunay-Weber: Overgrowth of extremity
  - Kasabach-Merritt: Hemangioma with consumption coagulopathy

Pulmonary Arteriovenous Fistula
- Part of hereditary hemorrhagic telangiectasia (Osler-Weber-Rendu)
- Leads to arterial hypoxemia due to intrapulmonary shunting

Coronary Arteriovenous Fistula
- If left coronary originates from pulmonary artery
- Left to right shunt via fistulous connection between right and left coronary arteries leads to volume overload and myocardial ischemia

Pathology

General
- Embryology
  - Persistence of primitive intracranial vascular connections, leading to dilatation of prosencephalic vein ~ great cerebral vein of Galen
- Pathophysiology
  - Extracardiac left to right shunt
  - Congestive heart failure to high cardiac output
  - Steal phenomenon of blood from normal vascular territory (cerebral white matter, kidneys, intestine)
- Epidemiology
  - Rare, < 1% of all congenital cardiovascular lesions

Clinical Issues

Presentation
- Large prenatal shunt: In utero congestive heart failure → hydrops fetalis
- High-output congestive heart failure in neonate
- Characteristic continuous murmur over the skull

Natural History
- Death from intractable congestive heart failure without treatment

Treatment
- Medical treatment for congestive heart failure
- Surgery has many complications
- Recent improvement in survival with transcatheter embolization and gamma-knife radiosurgery with stereotactic MRI targeting

Prognosis
- Guarded due to often-associated ischemic brain damage
- Determined by treatment complications

Selected References
1. Bothne A et al: Vein of Galen vascular malformations in infants: clinical, radiological and therapeutic aspect. Eur Radiol 7: 1252-8, 1997
2. Westra SJ et al: Pediatric intracranial vascular malformations: evaluation of treatment results with color Doppler US. Radiology 186: 775-83, 1993
3. Vogl TJ et al: MR angiography in children with cerebral neurovascular diseases: findings in 31 cases. Am J Roentgenol 159: 817-23, 1992

AV Malformation, Brain

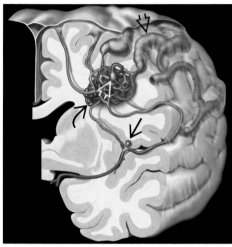

Coronal graphic depicts AV malformation (AVM). Note tightly packed nidus (curved arrow) with intranidal aneurysm (open white arrow), "pedicle" aneurysm (black arrow), and venous varices (open black arrow).

Key Facts
- Most common symptomatic cerebral vascular malformation (CVM)
- AVMs have dysregulated angiogenesis, undergo continued vascular remodeling

Imaging Findings
General Features
- Tightly packed mass of enlarged vascular channels
- No normal brain inside
- Best diagnostic sign = "bag of black worms" (flow voids) with minimal/no mass effect on MR

CT Findings
- NECT (may be normal with very small AVM)
  - Iso/hyperdense serpentine vessels
  - Ca++ in 25-30%
  - Variable hemorrhage
- CECT: Strong enhancement

MR Findings
- Varies with flow rate, direction, presence/age of hemorrhage
- "Honeycomb" of "flow voids"
- Nidus contains little or no normal brain tissue

Other Modality Findings
- DSA
  - Delineates internal angioarchitecture (superselective best)
  - Findings
    - Little or no mass effect
    - Enlarged arteries
    - Nidus of tightly packed vessels
    - AV shunt ("early draining vein")
- CTA/MRA
  - Helpful for gross depiction of flow, post-embo/XRT

AV Malformation, Brain

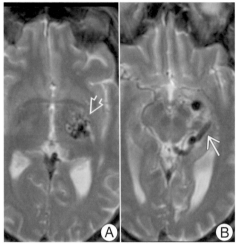

(A) T2W image shows nidus of AVM (open arrow) involving anterior thalamus and posterior limb of internal capsule, i.e., "eloquent brain"; the diameter is 2 cm. (B) Central draining vein (arrow). (All three are used in Spetzler-Martin scoring).

- o 3D contrast-enhanced studies improve delineation

Differential Diagnosis
Patent AVM vs. Glioblastoma (GBM) with AV Shunting
- GBM enhances, has mass effect
- Some parenchyma between vessels
Thrombosed ("Cryptic") AVM Versus
- Cavernous angioma
- Calcified neoplasm
- Oligodendroglioma
- Low-grade astrocytoma

Pathology
General
- General Path Comments
  - o 85% supratentorial; 15% posterior fossa
  - o Sporadic AVMs are solitary
- Genetics
  - o No specific mutations for sporadic AVMs
  - o Multiple AVMs (2% of cases)
    - HHT 1 (chromosome 9, 12 mutations)
    - Cerebral AV metameric syndromes (Wyburn-Mason) have orbit/ maxillofacial, intracranial AVMs
- Etiology-Pathogenesis
  - o Old: Retention of primitive embryonic vascular network?
  - o New: Dysregulated angiogenesis
    - VEGFs, receptors mediate endothelial proliferation, migration
    - Cytokine receptors mediate vascular maturation, remodeling
- Epidemiology
  - o Prevalence of sporadic AVMs = .04-.52%

AV Malformation, Brain

Gross Pathologic or Surgical Features
- Central nidus plus arterial feeders, venous outflow

Microscopic Features (Wide Phenotypic Spectrum)
- Feeding arteries, draining veins
  - Mature vessels (may have some wall thickening)
- Nidus
  - Thin-walled dysplastic vessels (no capillary bed)
    - Lack intact tight junctions, subendothelial support
    - Loss of normal contractile properties
  - Conglomeration of numerous AV shunts
  - No normal brain (may have some gliosis)
- Associated abnormalities
  - Flow-related aneurysm on feeding artery 10-15%
  - Intranidal "aneurysm" > 50%
  - Hemorrhage, +/- Ca++

Staging or Grading Criteria (Spetzler-Martin)
- Size
  - Small (< 3 cm)   1
  - Medium (3-6 cm)   2
  - Large (> 6 cm)   3
- Location
  - Noneloquent   0
  - Eloquent   1
- Venous drainage
  - Superficial only   0
  - Deep   1

Clinical Issues
Presentation
- Peak presentation = 20-40y (25% by age 15)
  - Hemorrhage 50%
  - Seizures 25%
  - Neurologic deficit 20-25%

Natural History
- Hemorrhage 2-4%/year, cumulative
- Spontaneous obliteration rare (1-3% of cases)

Treatment & Prognosis
- Embolization, radiosurgery, surgery

Selected References
1. Warren DJ et al: Cerebral arteriovenous malformations: Comparison of novel MRA techniques and conventional catheter angiography. Neurosurg 48: 973-83, 2001
2. Uranishi R et al: Vascular smooth muscle cell differentiation in human cerebral vascular malformations. Neurosurg 49: 671-80, 2001
3. Berman MF et al: The epidemiology of brain arteriovenous malformations. Neurosurg 47: 389-97, 2000

Venous Angioma

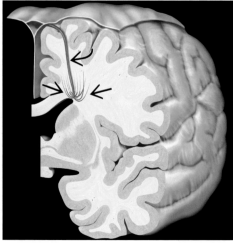

Coronal graphic depicts venous "angioma." Note upside-down umbrella appearance of prominent medullary veins ("Medusa head", black arrows) and single transcortical collector vein (curved arrow) draining into superior sagittal sinus (SSS).

Key Facts
- Venous angioma (VA) consists of angiogenically mature elements, represent anatomic variants of normal venous drainage (also called "developmental venous anomalies")
- Most VAs are asymptomatic
- VAs may be histologically mixed (cavernous malformation)

Imaging Findings
General Features
- Umbrella-like collection of enlarged medullary (white matter) veins
- Near ventricle (frontal horn, fourth ventricle most common sites)
- Large "collector" vein drains into dural sinus or deep ependymal vein
- Best diagnostic sign = "**Medusa head**" (dilated white matter veins)
CT Findings
- NECT: Usually normal
- CECT: Numerous linear or dot-like enhancing foci
  - Converge on single enlarged tubular draining vein
    - Occasionally seen as linear structure in a single slice
    - More often appears as well-circumscribed, round/ovoid enhancing areas on sequential sections
MR Findings
- Variable signal depending on size, flow rate
  - "Flow void" on T1, T2WI
- Strong enhancement
- Stellate, tubular vessels converge on **collector vein**
- Collector vein drains into dural sinus/ependymal vein
- +/- Hemorrhage (from co-existing cavernous malformation)
Other Modality Findings
- DSA
  - Arterial phase normal

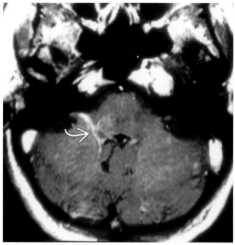

38-year-old woman with multiple sclerosis had venous angioma (curved arrow) incidentally noted near fourth ventricle.

- o Capillary phase
  - Usually normal
  - Rarely VAs may have prominent vascular blush, A-V shunt
- o Venous phase: "Medusa head" (or "caput medusa")

Differential Diagnosis
Vascular Neoplasm (e.g., GBM)
- Enlarged medullary veins
- Mass effect, usually enhances
Dural Sinus Occlusion With Venous Stasis
- Sinus thrombosis
- Medullary veins enlarge as collateral drainage
Demyelinating Disease (Rare)
- Active demyelination with prominent medullary veins

Pathology
General
- General Path Comments
  - o Most common cerebral vascular malformation at autopsy
- Genetics
  - o Mutations in chromosomes 1, 9
    - Encode for surface cell receptors
    - Tie-2 mutation results in missense activation, familial multiorgan venous malformations
  - o Some inherited as autosomal dominant
- Embryology
  - o Persistence of large embryonic white matter veins
- Etiology-Pathogenesis
  - o Do not express growth factors
  - o Express structural proteins of mature angiogenesis

- o May represent extreme anatomic variant of otherwise normal venous drainage
- Epidemiology
  - o 60% of cerebral vascular malformations
  - o 2.5-9% prevalence on contrast-enhanced MR scans
  - o Usually solitary
- Associated abnormalities
  - o Blue rubber bleb nevus syndrome
  - o Sinus pericranii
  - o Other cutaneous head and neck venous malformations
  - o Sulcation-gyration disorders

Gross Pathologic or Surgical Features
- Radially oriented dilated medullary veins
- Separated by normal brain
- Enlarged transcortical or subependymal draining vein

Microscopic Features
- Enlarged but otherwise normal veins
- Normal brain without gliosis
- 20% have mixed histology, may hemorrhage if downstream cavernous malformation

Clinical Issues
Presentation
- Usually **asymptomatic**, discovered incidentally at imaging
- Uncommon
  - o Headache
  - o Seizure (if associated with cortical dysplasia)
  - o Hemorrhage with focal neurologic deficit (if associated with cavernous malformation)

Natural History
- Hemorrhage risk 0.15% per lesion-year, increased if
  - o Stenosis or thrombosis of draining vein
  - o Co-existing cavernous malformation

Treatment & Prognosis
- Solitary VA: None (attempt at removal may cause venous infarction)
- Histologically mixed VA: Determined by co-existing lesion

Selected References
1. Kilic T et al: Expression of structural proteins and angiogenic factors in cerebrovascular anomalies. Neurosurg 46: 1179-92, 2000
2. Komiyama M et al: Venous angiomas with arteriovenous shunts. Neurosurg 44: 1328-35, 1999
3. Naff NJ et al: A longitudinal study of patients with venous malformations. Neurol 50: 1709-14, 1998

Cavernous Malformation

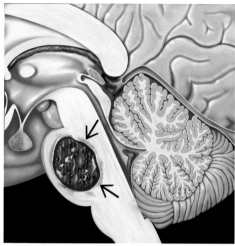

Sagittal graphic depicts typical cavernous malformation, shown here in the pons. Locules of blood with fluid-fluid levels, hemorrhage in different stages, and some flocculent Ca++ are present. Hemosiderin rim surrounds the lesion (arrows).

Key Facts
- CM (cavernous "angioma") should not be confused with cavernous **hem**angioma (true vasoproliferative neoplasm)
- CM = most common angiographically "occult" vascular malformation
- CMs exhibit range of dynamic behaviors (enlargement, regression, **de novo** formation)
- Familial CMs at high risk for hemorrhage, forming new lesions

Imaging Findings
General Features
- Discrete, lobulated mass
- Bleeding, variable maturation of blood products
- Best diagnostic sign = "**popcorn ball**" with complete hemosiderin rim
CT Findings
- Negative in 30-50%
- Well-delineated round/ovoid hyperdense lesion, usually < 3 cm
- Surrounding brain usually appears normal
- No mass effect unless recent hemorrhage
- Little/no enhancement
MR Findings
- Variable, depending on hemorrhage/stage
- Large acute hemorrhage may obscure more typical features of CM
- Reticulated "popcorn-like" lesion most typical
    - Mixed signal core, complete hemosiderin rim
    - Locules of blood with fluid-fluid levels
    - Susceptibility effect (lesion "blooms" on T2WI, T2* scans)
    - Minimal or no enhancement (may show associated venous malformation)
- If > 3 lesions, numerous punctate hypointense foci ("black dots") on GRE scans most common finding (even darker on b = 0 image from diffusion study)

Cavernous Malformation

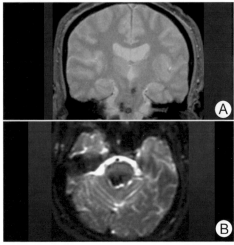

(A) Coronal GRE demonstrates multiple punctate pontine areas of low signal corresponding to cavernous angiomas. (B) Axial b=0 image through pons from diffusion study shows even greater signal loss.

Other Modality Findings
- DSA
  - Negative ("angiographically occult vascular malformation")
    - CMs have slow intralesional flow without AV shunting
  - Avascular mass effect if large or acute hemorrhage
  - +/- Associated other malformation (e.g., VM)
  - Rare: Venous pooling, contrast "blush"

Differential Diagnosis
"Popcorn Ball" Lesion
- AVM (edema, mass effect, often single blood product)
- Hemorrhagic neoplasm (incomplete hemosiderin rim, disordered evolution of blood products, strong enhancement)
- Calcified neoplasm (e.g., oligodendroglioma; usually shows some enhancement)
Multiple "Black Dots"
- Old trauma (diffuse axonal injury, contusions)
- Hypertensive microbleeds (history of longstanding hypertension)
- Amyloid angiopathy (elderly, demented, white matter disease)
- Capillary telangiectasias (faint "brush-like" enhancement)

Pathology
General
- Genetics
  - Multiple (familial) CM syndrome
    - Autosomal dominant, variable penetrance
    - Mutation in chromosomes 3,7q (KRIT1 mutation at CCM1)
- Etiology-Pathogenesis-Pathophysiology
  - CMs are angiogenically immature lesions with endothelial proliferation, increased neoangiogenesis

- o VEGF, βFGF, TGF α expressed
- o Receptors (e.g., Flk-1) upregulated
- Epidemiology
  - o Approximate prevalence 0.5%; M = F
  - o 75% occur as solitary, sporadic lesion
  - o Probably due to cavernous transformation from venous angioma
  - o 10%-30% multiple, familial

Gross Pathologic or Surgical Features
- Discrete, lobulated, bluish-purple ("mulberry-like") nodule
- Pseudocapsule of gliotic, hemosiderin-stained brain

Microscopic Features
- Thin-walled epithelial-lined spaces
- Embedded in collagenous matrix
- Hemorrhage in different stages of evolution
- +/- Ca++
- Does not contain normal brain
- May be histologically mixed (venous malformation most common)

Clinical Issues

Presentation
- Peak presentation = 40-60y but may present in childhood
- Symptoms
  - o Seizure 50%
  - o Neurologic deficit 25% (may be progressive)
  - o 20% asymptomatic

Natural History
- Broad range of dynamic behavior (may progress, enlarge, regress)
- **De novo** lesions may develop
- Propensity for repeated intralesional hemorrhages
  - o Sporadic = 0.25-0.7%/year
  - o Familial = approximately 1% per lesion per year
  - o Risk factor for future hemorrhage = previous hemorrhage
  - o Rehemorrhage rate high initially, decreases after 2-3 years

Selected References
1. Sure U et al: Endothelial proliferation, neoangiogenesis, and potential de novo generation of cerebrovascular malformations. J Neurosurg 94: 972-7, 2001
2. Bruneread L et al: Familial form of intracranial cavernous angioma. Radiology 214: 209-16, 2000
3. Dillon WP: Cryptic vascular malformations: controversies in terminology, diagnosis, pathophysiology, and treatment. AJNR 18: 1839-46,1997

Capillary Telangiectasia

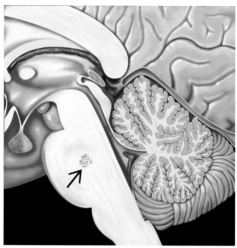

Sagittal graphic depicts pontine capillary telangiectasia (arrow). Note enlarged capillaries with normal brain between the dilated vessels.

Key Facts
- Most capillary telangiectasias (CT)s are discovered incidentally at imaging or autopsy
- Clinically benign (unless histologically mixed with other malformation such as cavernous or venous malformation)
- CTs contain normal brain

Imaging Findings
General Features
- Small, poorly-demarcated lesion(s)
- Consists of dilated capillaries
- Contains normal brain
- No gross hemorrhage
- Midbrain, pons, medulla, spinal cord most common sites
- Best diagnostic sign = ill-defined lesion with faint "**brush-like**" **enhancement**

CT Findings
- Usually normal

MR Findings
- Solitary lesion
  - ○ T1WI usually normal
  - ○ 50% are hyperintense on T2WI, FLAIR
  - ○ May be hypointense on T2* scan (slow intralesional blood flow permits desaturation of oxy- to deoxyhemoglobin)
  - ○ Faint stippled or brush-like enhancement with small punctate and linear/branching vessels
  - ○ Up to 2/3 have enlarged collecting vein (may be mixed with venous malformation)
- Multifocal hypointensities on T2WI, GRE scans ("black dots")

DSA/MRA/CTA Findings
- Negative unless mixed malformation (e.g., venous)

Capillary Telangiectasia

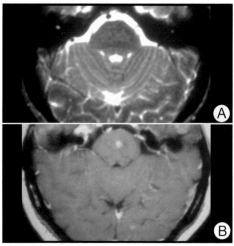

MRI of capillary telangiectasia. The lesion is inapparent on T2WI (A) and shows as central pontine enhancement on enhanced T1WI (B).

Differential Diagnosis
Metastasis
- Usually enhances strongly
- Location (gray-white junction; pons/cerebellum rare)

Cavernous Malformation
- Blood locules with fluid-fluid levels
- Abnormalities in adjacent brain (e.g., hemosiderin rim)
- Mixed capillary/cavernous or capillary venous malformation

Pathology
General
- Etiology-Pathogenesis
  - Sporadic CTs: Unknown
  - May develop as complication of radiation (usually whole brain, often for leukemia)
- Epidemiology
  - 15-20% of all intracranial vascular malformations

Gross Pathologic or Surgical Features
- Rarely identified unless unusually large (up to 2 cm reported) or hemorrhage (from other vascular malformation) present

Microscopic Features
- Numerous dilated but histologically normal capillaries
- Normal brain between enlarged capillary channels
- Uncomplicated CTs have no gliosis, hemorrhage, Ca++
- May be histologically mixed (CM most common)
  - Blood products

Clinical Issues
Presentation
- Rarely symptomatic, usually discovered incidentally

Capillary Telangiectasia

- Rare
  - Headache
  - Vertigo, tinnitus
  - Cranial neuropathy

Natural History
- Clinically quiescent unless histologically mixed
- No change in size or configuration

Treatment & Prognosis
- None

Selected References
1. Castillo M et al: MR imaging and histologic features of capillary telangiectasia of the basal ganglia. AJNR 22: 1553-5, 2001
2. Kuker W et al: Presumed capillary telangiectasia of the pons. Eur Radiol 10: 945-50, 2000
3. Huddle DC et al: Clinically aggressive diffuse capillary telangiectasia of the brain stem. AJNR 20: 1674-7, 1999

Pediatric/Young Adult Stroke

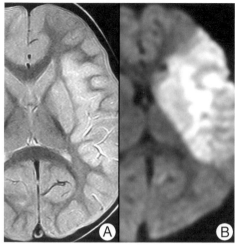

2-year-old with spontaneous left common carotid artery dissection and left MCA infarct. (A) Proton density weighted image shows hyperintensity in left MCA territory. (B) Diffusion image is positive, indicating acute infarct.

Key Facts
- Pediatric stroke etiologies extremely varied
- Neonate/infant: R-L cardiac shunt, birth trauma
- < 15 y: Prothrombic states cause 20-50% of arterial ischemic strokes
  - 33-99% sinovenous thrombosis
- > 15 y: Dissection, atherothrombosis, more "traditional" risk factors

Imaging Findings
General Features
- Similar to adults
CT Findings
- Similar to adults
- Look for clues to stroke etiology
  - Basal ganglia Ca++ (MELAS, cranial irradiation)
  - Vascular anomaly (check presence/size of carotid canal)
  - Pre-existing atrophy (SLE, other collagen-vascular disease)
  - Enhancing "dots" in basal ganglia ("moya-moya" collaterals)
MR Findings
- Similar to adults
- Look for clues to stroke etiology
  - Stigmata of neurocutaneous disorder (e.g., NF-1)
  - Midline malformations
  - Metabolic disease (e.g., MELAs, Leigh's)
- DWI: Acute restriction + chronic changes (new stroke superimposed on old, e.g., sickle-cell, moya moya)
Imaging Recommendations
- Screening CECT may give early clue to
  - Perfusion of normal vs. "drop out" of ischemic tissue
  - Circle of Willis patency
  - Presence of sinovenous occlusion

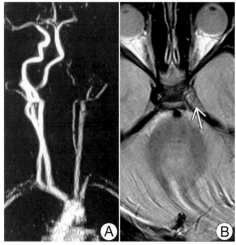

2-year-old with spontaneous left ICA dissection and MCA infarct. (A) 2D TOF MRA demonstrates absent left ICA. (B) Proton density weighted axial image does not show flow void in expected position of left internal carotid artery (arrow), indicating occlusion.

- MR/MRA/MRV
- DWI

Differential Diagnosis
Nonischemic Causes of Acute Childhood Hemiparesis
- Todd's paralysis following seizure
- ADEM (acute disseminated encephalomyelitis)
Newly Noticed Hemiparesis
- Perinatal infarct
- Congenital anomaly (i.e., schizencephaly)
- Caution
  - o Hemiparesis sometimes noticed only when child old enough to walk/ use hands purposefully
  - o Brain anomaly/perinatal stroke may seem "acute" at 9 to 18 mo

Pathology
General
- Etiology-Pathogenesis-Pathophysiology (multifactorial)
  - o Cardiac (embolism, valve anomaly, left atrial myxoma)
  - o Congenital prothrombic disorders
    - ▪ Resistance to: Activated protein C
    - ▪ Deficiencies of: Antithrombin, protein S or C
    - ▪ Presence of: Factor V-Leiden, anti-cardiolipin/anti-phospholipid antibodies, lupus anticoagulant, etc.
  - o Acquired prothrombic disorders
    - ▪ Hyperlipidemia, polycythemia, iron deficiency anemia, platelet disorders, leukemia, chemotherapy-related
  - o Other inherited disorders

- Skull base anomaly with absent carotid canal (e.g., Morning-glory syndrome with colobomas, vasculopathy, pituitary malfunction, sphenopharyngeal encephalocele)
- Neurocutaneous syndrome: NF-1, tuberous sclerosis
- Vasculopathies: Cerebral autosomal dominant arteriopathy with subcortical infarcts and leukoencephalopathy (CADASIL), cerebral autosomal recessive arteriopathy with subcortical infarcts and leokoencephacopathy (CARASIL), sickle-cell anemia
- Metabolic: MELAS, homocystinuria, premature aging (progeria)
  - o Other acquired disorders
    - Migraine, dissection
    - Non-accidental injury
    - Vasculopathies: Chickenpox; isolated CNS angiitis; systemic angiitis (Kawasaki, Takayasu, polyarteritis nodosa, Behçet's); moyamoya phenomenon (idiopathic or secondary)
    - Any progressive vasculopathy $\Rightarrow$ moya-moya-like radiology findings
    - Teen/young adult: Add "street" drugs, oral contraceptives
    - Young adult: Add atheroembolic, cigarette smoking, diabetes

Staging or Grading Criteria
- Moya-moya 1-6
  - o 1 = stenosis distal ICA
  - o 2-5 = opening then closing of basal collaterals
  - o 6= dependence on transdural collaterals

Clinical Issues
Presentation
- Infant
  - o Seizure
  - o Poor feeding, developmental delay
- Older children: Depends upon size, vascular distribution

Treatment & Prognosis
- Treat etiologic factor(s)
- Anticoagulation (aspirin/heparin/Coumadin)
- Immunosuppression (autoimmune)
- Symptomatic moya-moya (synangiosis?)

Selected References
1. Chan AK et al: Prothrombotic disorders and ischemic stroke in children. Semin Pediatr Neurol 7: 301-8, 2000
2. Williams LS et al: Subtypes of ischemic stroke in children and young adults. Neurology 49: 1541-5, 1997
3. Giroud M et al: Stroke in children under 16 years of age. Clinical and etiological difference with adults. Acta Neurol Scand 96: 401-6, 1997

Sickle Cell Anemia

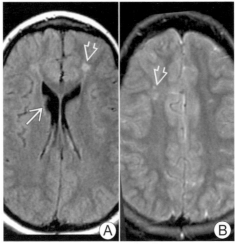

14-year-old boy with sickle cell anemia & multiple prior strokes (open arrows). (A) Axial FLAIR shows R caudate head encephalomalacia (arrow) from prior infarct. This reflects stenosis of R recurrent artery of Huebner & proximal M1 segment lenticulostriates. (B) Axial PDWI shows white matter infarcts (open arrows).

Key Facts
- Primary cause of stroke in children of African-American origin
  - Stroke incidence decreased if Hgb S kept to less than 30% by transfusion (but need initial ischemic event to initiate therapy)
  - Use MRI to document previous ischemic events
- Key imaging findings
  - Stenosis of distal ICA and proximal circle of Willis (COW) vessels
  - Moya-moya, i.e., lenticulostriate collaterals
  - Cortical and deep white matter infarcts
    - Often in distal watershed between ACA and MCA territories
- Caveat: Cognitive impairment does **not** correlate with imaging findings

Imaging Findings
General Features
- Best imaging clue: Narrowing of the distal ICAs leading to moya-moya
CT Findings
- NECT: Focal encephalomalacia due to cortical infarction
- CECT: Punctate enhancement in basal ganglia due to moya-moya collaterals (better seen on CEMR)
- CTA: Stenosis distal ICA and proximal COW vessels
MR Findings
- FLAIR, PDWI, or T2WI: Hyperintensity and local atrophy due to gliosis from cortical or deep white matter infarction
- MRA
  - Aneurysms in atypical locations
  - Stenosis of distal ICA and proximal COW vessels
    - Caveat: Turbulent dephasing due to anemia and rapid flow can stimulate stenosis on bright blood MRA
    - Suggestion: Use lowest possible TE for bright blood MRA or use black blood MRA if stenosis suspected

Sickle Cell Anemia

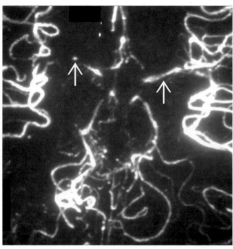

3D MRA in a 7-year-old boy with sickle cell anemia and narrowing MCAs, right > left (arrows).

- MRA source images: Multiple dots in basal ganglia due to moya-moya
- Contrast-enhanced T1WI: Vascular stasis and leptomeningeal collaterals in MCA territory with proximal MCA stenosis
- Diffusion/perfusion imaging: Decreased diffusion and perfusion during acute stroke

Other Modality Findings
- TCD: Hyperdynamic flow in MCA due to proximal stenosis
- DSA: Stenosis of distal ICA and proximal COW vessels, fusiform aneurysms, moya-moya collaterals and EC-IC collaterals
  - o Risk of stroke higher than in other populations
  - o Hydrate, transfuse and sedate before catheter study

Imaging Recommendations
- MRI to exclude previous infarcts and short TE bright blood MRA or black blood MRA to exclude distal ICA stenosis and moya-moya collaterals

Differential Diagnosis

Vasculitis
- Infectious, autoimmune or substance abuse etiologies
- Classic imaging findings: Cortical and deep white matter infarcts and parenchymal hemorrhage

Connective Tissue Disorders
- Marfan, Ehlers-Danlos, homocystinuria
- Progressive arterial narrowing and occlusion

Pathology

General
- Initial endothelial injury from abnormal adherence of sickled erythrocytes
- Subsequently internal elastic lamina fragmentation and degeneration of muscularis result in large vessel vasculopathy and aneurysm formation
  - o May be reversed with transfusion
- Genetics: Homozygous for Hgb S

Sickle Cell Anemia

- Etiology-Pathogenesis
  - Heterozygous Hgb S affords increased resistance to malaria (hence prevalence)
- Epidemiology
  - SS disease found primarily in African-Americans and their descendents
  - Homozygous SS leads to sickling and vascular occlusion ("crisis")

Gross Pathologic or Surgical Features
- Bone, brain, renal and splenic infarcts; hepatomegaly

Microscopic Features
- Severe anemia with sickled cells on smear
- Vascular occlusions due to masses of sickled cells

Clinical Issues

Presentation
- Hgb S found in 10% of African-Americans
- **Stroke** in **African-American children**
  - 75% are ischemic, 25% are hemorrhage
  - 17-26% of all patients with sickle cell anemia
  - Cognitive impairment does not correlate with MR findings
- Bone infarcts, avascular necrosis during crisis
- Osteomyelitis, especially Salmonella
- Gross hematuria from renal papillary necrosis and ulceration
- Splenic infarction from exposure to high altitude, e.g., flying
- Infections common, especially pneumococcus after splenic infarction

Natural History
- Unrelenting, severe hemolytic anemia beginning at a few months of age after Hgb S replaces Hgb F (fetal)
- Repeated ischemic events leading to strokes with worsening motor and intellectual deficits

Treatment
- Repeated transfusions to keep Hgb S less than 30% decreases both incidence of stroke and intimal hyperplasia in COW vessels
- Folic acid for anemia
- Hydration and oxygenation during crises

Prognosis
- Poor for homozygous SS disease without transfusions
- Usually live to adulthood albeit with complications

Selected References
1. Oyesiku NM et al: Intracranial aneurysms in sickle-cell anemia: clinical features and pathogenesis. J Neurosurg 75: 356-63, 1991
2. Wiznitzer M et al: Diagnosis of cerebrovascular disease in sickle cell anemia by magnetic resonance angiography. J Pediatr 117(4): 551-5, 1990
3. Rothman SM et al: Sickle cell anemia and central nervous system infarction: a neuropathological study. Ann Neurol 20: 684-90, 1986

Atherosclerosis, Intracranial

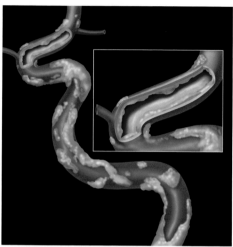

Graphic depiction of atherosclerotic plaques causing luminal narrowing, particularly at carotid siphon (insert).

Key Facts
- Atherosclerosis is a systemic, multifactorial disease
- Intracranial atherosclerosis is
  - Third most common cause of thromboembolic stroke
  - After carotid and cardiac sources
- Classic imaging appearance
  - Stenotic intracranial vessel on angiogram
  - Usually involves
    - Proximal circle of Willis (COW)
    - Distal basilar or internal carotid arteries

Imaging Findings
General Features
- Best imaging clue: Stenotic intracranial artery on angiogram
CT Findings
- NECT: Calcified artery
- CTA: Calcifications in wall and narrowed lumen
MR Findings
- T1WI: Decreased flow void in expected position of artery
- T2WI: Decreased flow void in expected position of artery
- MRA: Focal stenosis, ectasia or irregularity on 3D TOF MRA or MOTSA
  - Caveat 1: Contralateral vessel must be normal caliber throughout
  - Caveat 2: MRA tends to overestimate stenosis
Other Modality Findings
- Trans-Cranial Doppler (TCD): Increased velocities
- DSA: Focal stenosis, luminal irregularities, thrombosis, occlusion
  - Less commonly: Ectasia and elongation, serpentine aneurysms
Imaging Recommendations
- MRA (MOTSA) of brain followed by more invasive DSA

Atherosclerosis, Intracranial

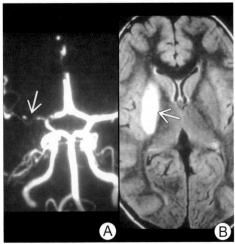

(A) Stenosis of M1 segment of right MCA (arrow). (B) Proton density weighted image demonstrates infarct in right basal ganglia (arrow) due to (A).

Differential Diagnosis

Vasculitis
- Usually just involves smaller (tertiary) branches
- More likely to be associated with hemorrhage

Arteritis
- Usually painful
- Elevated ESR, autoimmune parameters

Spasm From SAH
- Associated SAH (on NECT or FLAIR MRI)

Moya-Moya
- Usually distal ICAs and proximal COW with relative sparing of basilar

Pathology

General
- General Path Comments
  - Intracranial atherosclerosis associated with atherosclerosis of carotids, coronaries, aorta, renal arteries, iliofemoral system
- Anatomy
  - Most often involves arterial bifurcations, e.g., ICA and basilar
  - May involve distal arterioles leading to vasculitis pattern of alternating stenosis and dilatation
- Etiology-Pathogenesis
  - Probably multiple etiologies; the main three are
    - Lipid Hypothesis: High plasma LDL leads to LDL-cholesterol deposition in intima
    - Response to Injury Hypothesis: Focal endothelial change or intimal injury leads to platelet aggregation and plaque formation
    - Unifying Hypothesis: Endothelial injury leads to increased permeability of LDL: Plaques grow by formation of thrombi on plaque surface and transendothelial leakage of plasma lipids

Atherosclerosis, Intracranial

- Epidemiology
  - More common in Western countries

Gross Pathologic Features
- Earliest macroscopic finding: Intimal fatty streaks
- Fibrous atheromatous plaques contain
  - Smooth muscle cells, monocytes, other leukocytes
  - Connective tissue: Collagen, elastic fibers, proteoglycans
  - Intra- and extracellular lipid deposits
  - Angiogenesis produces new capillaries at plaque periphery
    - Leads to intraplaque hemorrhage and ulceration
    - Hemorrhage leads to dystrophic ferrocalcinosis (seen more as calcification on CT and as iron on MR)
- Arterial narrowing due to atherosclerotic plaque
  - Becomes flow limiting beyond 70% stenosis (based on diameter ratios)
  - Ischemic symptoms depend on presence of collaterals
    - Slow occlusion generally leads to multiple collaterals, fewer symptoms
    - Rapid occlusion (from thrombosis or artery-to-artery embolus): Not enough time for collaterals to develop, infarct likely
- Arterial irregularity due to disruption of endothelial surface may form thrombogenic surface leading to thrombosis or artery-to-artery embolus

Microscopic Features
- Earliest findings
  - Lipid deposition and cellular reaction in intimal layer of arterial wall
- Later findings in atherosclerotic plaques
  - Lipid core
  - Fibrous cap (the thicker, the more stable and less likely to rupture)

Clinical Issues

Presentation
- **Plaque rupture** usually leads to **stroke**
- Vascular stenosis leads to stuttering ischemic symptoms due to intermittent thrombosis

Natural History
- Progressive disease unless treated aggressively

Treatment
- Low saturated fat and cholesterol diet; exercise (probably secondary)
- Cholesterol lowering drugs (primary source of cholesterol so main treatment)
- Plaque stabilization (via "statin" drugs) may decrease stroke
- Angioplasty (? ready for prime time)

Prognosis
- Poor without treatment
- Better with treatment

Selected References
1. Osborn AG: Atherosclerosis and carotid stenosis. in: Diagnostic cerebral angiography (2nd Ed), Lippincott Williams and Wilkins, Philadelphia, 359-79, 1999
2. Garcia JH et al: Carotid atherosclerosis: definition, pathogenesis, and clinical significance. Neuroimaging Clinics of North America 6: 801-10, 1996
3. Consigny PJ: Pathogenesis of atherosclerosis. AJR 164: 553-8, 1995

Atherosclerosis, Extracranial

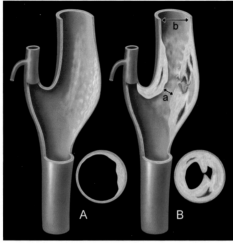

Graphic depiction of mild and severe carotid atherosclerotic vascular disease (ASVD). (A) Earliest signs of ASVD are "fatty streaks" and slight intimal thickening. (B) Severe stenosis with intraplaque hemorrhage, ulceration and platelet emboli are shown. NASCET calculation: % stenosis = (b-a)/b x 100.

Key Facts
- Atherogenesis is a complex, multifactorial process
- Carotid bifurcation is the most common site in head, neck
- Spectrum of pathology includes ectasia, stenosis, ulceration with platelet thrombi, embolization + silent or symptomatic infarction

Imaging Findings
General Features
- Best diagnostic sign = narrowing of proximal internal carotid artery (ICA)
- **70**% diameter narrowing = NASCET criterion for carotid endarterectomy

CT Findings
- Ca++ in vessel wall (ICA, basilar artery (BA) most common sites)
- Ectasia, tortuosity
- Fusiform dilatation
- Stenosis, occlusion (CTA)

MR Findings
- Lumen narrowed, wall thickened
- Absent "flow void" (occurs with occlusion, very slow flow)
- Stenosis (severe narrowing causes "flow gap" on unenhanced TOF MRA)

Other Modality Findings
- U/S
  - Plaque characteristics and clinical correlation
    - Hypoechoic plaques are independent risk factor for stroke
    - Acoustic shadowing correlates with ischemic stroke
  - Increased intima/media thickness = sign of early atherosclerosis vascular disease (ASVD) (but clinical significance controversial)
- DSA
  - Plaque surface irregularity associated with increased stroke risk at all degrees of stenosis (presumed ulceration)

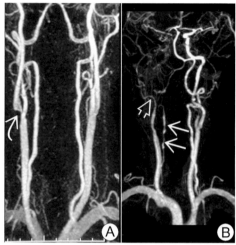

Two patients with MRA demonstrating carotid ASVD. (A) High-grade stenosis at origin of right internal carotid artery (RICA) (curved arrow). (B) Complete occlusion of RICA (open arrow) and multiple stenoses of right vertebral artery (arrows). Both patients had TIAs.

- o Detects "tandem" (siphon) stenoses, depicts collateral circulation
- [111]In platelet scintigraphy
  - o Detects thrombotic complications in carotid plaque

Imaging Recommendations
- U/S as initial screening procedure
- CTA/CE - MRA
- Consider DSA prior to endarterectomy

Differential Diagnosis

Dissection
- Spares bulb
- Usually smoother, longer narrowing; no Ca++
- Neck pain, Horner's syndrome

Pathology

General
- General Path Comments
  - o Severity of vessel narrowing is important
  - o Detection of "vulnerable plaque" most important as it leads to rupture, local thrombus, potential for distal (artery-to-artery) embolization, and stroke; need to look for
    - ▪ Thickness of fibrous cap (thicker is more stable)
    - ▪ Size of lipid core (smaller is more stable)
- Genetics
  - o Probably multigenic
  - o Many specific polymorphisms identified
- Etiology-Pathogenesis-Pathophysiology
  - o ASVD development, progression is complex, multifactorial
    - ▪ Diet, genes
    - ▪ Mechanical factors (e.g., anatomic variations, wall shear stress)

- Role of infection (e.g., Helicobacter, Chlamydia), inflammation (activated endothelial cells, cytokine release) controversial, C-reactive protein elevation
- Epidemiology
  - Leading cause of morbidity, mortality in Western world
  - Ischemic stroke accounts for up to 40% of deaths in elderly
  - Cerebral infarcts occur in > 70% of patients with carotid occlusion
  - 90% of large, recent cerebral infarcts caused by thromboemboli
  - Lacunar infarcts correlate with both hypertension and ASVD

Gross Pathologic or Surgical Features
- Intimal "fatty streaks" early sign
- As disease progresses, fibrotic cap covers core of foam cells, necrotic debris, cholesterol

Microscopic Features
- Monocyte-derived macrophages, smooth muscle cells proliferate
- Become lipid-filled "foam cells"
- Neovascularity may cause intraplaque hemorrhage
- Ulceration may ensue, platelet adhesion/thrombi form

Clinical Issues
Presentation
- Variable
  - Can be asymptomatic
  - Bruit
  - Stroke
- Risk (stroke) increases with smoking, hypertension, diabetes, overweight, inferior socioeconomic circumstances

Natural History
- Progressive; significant stenosis may cause decreased perfusion
- Artery-to-artery emboli

Treatment & Prognosis
- Endarterectomy if carotid stenosis ≥ 70%

Selected References
1. Ameriso SF et al: Detection of Helicobacter pylori in human carotid atherosclerotic plaques. Stroke 32: 385-91, 2001
2. Shaaban AM et al: Wall shear stress and early atherosclerosis: A review. AJR 174: 1657-65, 2000
3. Ballotta E et al: Carotid plaque gross morphology and clinical presentation: A prospective study of 457 carotid artery specimens. J Surg Res 89: 78-84, 2000

Acute Ischemic Stroke

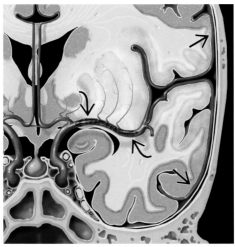

Coronal graphic depicts hyperacute stroke. Fresh thrombus (curved arrows) is seen in the proximal MCA. Retrograde flow through watershed collaterals is present (arrows). Note pallor, swelling of the basal ganglia and affected cortex with effaced gray-white matter interfaces.

Key Facts
- "Time is brain"
- Diffusion weighted imaging (DWI) should be performed before thrombolysis because
  - Diagnosis of stroke incorrect 20% of cases
  - Silent stroke > 3 hours old 10% of cases
  - No ischemic penumbra 20% of cases
- Imaging diagnosis, intervention key for salvaging "at risk" tissue

Imaging Findings
General Features
- Acute thrombus in cerebral vessel(s)
- Decreased perfusion within territory of occluded vessel
- Cytotoxic edema
- Best diagnostic signs: High signal on DWI
CT Findings (NECT)
- Hyperattenuating vessel
  - Hyperdense M1 MCA ("dense MCA sign") in 35-50%
  - "Dot sign" = occluded MCA branches in sylvian fissure
- Loss of gray-white matter differentiation within first 3 hours
  - Subtle findings present in 50-70% of cases
    - Lentiform nucleus obscured
    - Insular "ribbon" lost
- Parenchymal hypodensity
  - If > 1/3 MCA territory on initial CT, large lesion later
- Gyral swelling, sulcal effacement
- "Hemorrhagic transformation"
  - Delayed onset (24-48h)
  - Can be gross or petechial
  - 15-45% of cases on NECT

Acute Ischemic Stroke

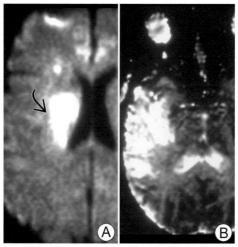

Acute right MCA infarct 7 hours post ictus. (A) DWI demonstrates hyperintensity in right basal ganglia (arrow) indicating acute infarct. (B) Perfusion imaging (mean transit time map) demonstrates larger abnormality corresponding to most of MCA territory. The difference between A and B is the "ischemic penumbra".

o Risk factors: Early CT signs of ischemic stroke, thromboembolic stroke, diabetes, decreased consciousness, thrombolysis

MR Findings
- Conventional sequences + in 70-80%
  o T1WI: Early cortical swelling, subtle loss of gray-white borders
  o T2WI: Hyperintensity in affected distribution
  o T1WI + contrast: Intravascular enhancement
- FLAIR:May be + (hyperintense) when other sequences normal
  o Intraarterial signal = early sign of major vessel occlusion
- DWI: Restricted diffusion (high signal), improves accuracy to 95%
- ADC: Evolves faster for thromboembolic vs. watershed infarct
  o Intermediate ADC = "at risk" tissue
  o Significantly reduced ADC = brain that will infarct
- PWI with rCBF (rCBV/MTT) map: Decreased perfusion
  o 75% are larger than lesion on DWI (difference is **"ischemic penumbra"** tissue, i.e., at risk for extension of infarct)
  o 25% of strokes only positive on PWI, not DWI

Other Modality Findings
- DSA: Vessel occlusion (cutoff, tapered, meniscus, tram-track), slow antegrade flow, retrograde collateral flow across watershed
- Triphasic perfusion CTA: Ischemic core, penumbra depicted
- TCD: Proximal occlusion in 70% of thrombolysis-eligible patients

Imaging Recommendations
- MRI (with FLAIR, DWI and PWI)
- DSA with thrombolysis in selected patients with acute ischemic stroke

Differential Diagnosis

Hyperdense Vessel Sign
- Normal (circulating blood is slightly hyperdense to brain)
- High hematocrit

- Microcalcification in vessel wall
- Diffuse cerebral edema makes vessels appear relatively hyperdense

Parenchymal Hypodensity
- Infiltrating neoplasm, inflammation (e.g., encephalitis)

Pathology
General
- Etiology-Pathogenesis-Pathophysiology
  - Early: Critical disturbance in cerebral blood flow (CBF)
    - Severely ischemic core has CBF < 6 ml/100g/min
    - Causes oxygen depletion, energy failure, terminal depolarization, ion homeostasis failure
    - Represents bulk of final infarct
    - Ischemic penumbra CBF between 7 and 20 ml/100g/min
  - Secondary changes include excitotoxicity, SD-like depolarizations, disturbance of ion homeostasis: "Glutamate cascade"
  - Evolution from ischemia to infarction depends on many factors (e.g., BP fluctuations, embolic fragmentation, reperfusion)
  - Delayed effects: Inflammation, apoptosis
- Epidemiology
  - Second most common worldwide cause of death
  - Major cause of long-term disability

Gross Pathologic or Surgical Features
- Acute thrombosis of major vessel
- Pale, swollen brain; gray-white matter boundaries "smudged"

Microscopic Features
- After 4h: Eosinophilic neurons with pyknotic nuclei
- 15-24h: Neutrophils invade; necrotic nuclei "eosinophilic ghosts"
- 2-3 days: Blood-derived phagocytes
- 1 week: Reactive astrocytosis, increased capillary density
- End result: Fluid-filled cavity lined by astrocytes

Clinical Issues
Presentation
- DDx stroke: Seizure (Todd's paralysis), migraine, inflammation

Natural History
- 60% improve over time without treatment
- "Malignant" MCA infarct (coma, death)
  - Up to 10% of all stroke patients
  - Fatal brain swelling with increased intracranial pressure

Treatment & Prognosis
- Thrombolysis improves outcome
- Patient selection = most important factor in treatment outcome
  - < 6h, lack of hemorrhage, < 1/3 MCA territory

Selected References
1. Parsons MW et al: Perfusion MRI maps in hyperacute stroke. Stroke 32: 1581-7, 2001
2. Huang I-J et al: Time course of cerebral infarction in the middle cerebral artery territory: Deep watershed versus territorial subtypes on diffusion-weighted MR images. Radiology 221: 35-42, 2001
3. Gaskill-Shipley MF: Routine CT evaluation of acute stroke. Neuroimag Clin N Amer 9: 411-22, 1999

Cerebral Amyloid Angiopathy

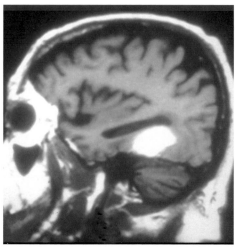

Early subacute hematoma in subcortical temporal lobe of elderly demented patient. T1WI demonstrates high signal indicating methemoglobin.

Key Facts
- Cerebral amyloid angiopathy (CAA) is common cause of "spontaneous" lobar hemorrhage in elderly
- CAA common in elderly patient with dementia (e.g., Alzheimer)

Imaging Findings
General Features
- **Superficial hemorrhages** involve cortex, subcortical white matter
- Best diagnostic sign = normotensive demented patient with
  - Lobar hemorrhage(s), different ages
  - Multifocal "black dots" on T2*WI

CT Findings
- NECT
  - Patchy or confluent cortical/subcortical hematoma with irregular borders, surrounding edema
  - Rare: Gyriform Ca++
- CECT
  - No enhancement

MR Findings
- T1WI
  - **Lobar hematoma** (signal varies with age of clot)
  - Generalized atrophy common (prominent ventricles, sulci)
- T2WI
  - Acute hematoma; 1/3 have old hemorrhages (lobar, petechial)
  - Focal or patchy/confluent WM disease in nearly 70%
  - Rare: Nonhemorrhagic diffuse encephalopathy with confluent WM hyperintensities
- T2*
  - Multifocal "**black dots**"
- Rare: CAA can cause focal, nonhemorrhagic mass(es), enhance, mimic neoplasm

Cerebral Amyloid Angiopathy

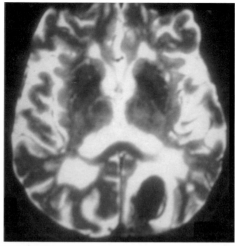

Same patient as the previous page. T2WI demonstrates low signal, indicating that red cells are still intact and that hematoma is in early subacute phase.

Other Modality Findings
- DSA: Normal or avascular mass effect

Imaging Recommendations
- Include T2*-weighted GRE sequence in patients > 60y

Differential Diagnosis
Hypertensive Microhemorrhages
- History of chronic hypertension (HTN)
- Deep structures (basal ganglia, thalami) > cortex, subcortical whitematter (WM)
- Often coexist with CAA

Ischemic Stroke With Microhemorrhage
- Multifocal hemosiderin deposits (10-15% of patients with ischemic stroke)
- Hemorrhagic lacunar infarcts

Multiple Vascular Malformations
- Cavernous, capillary malformations
  - Look for "locules" of blood with fluid-fluid levels
  - Capillary hemangiomas may show faint, "brush-like" enhancement

Other Causes of Multifocal "Black Dots"
- Traumatic axonal injury (history, location in corpus callosum)
- Hemorrhagic metastases (may enhance, location at gray-white junction)

Pathology
General
- General Path Comments
  - CNS amyloid can cause lobar hemorrhage (most common), microangiopathy, focal "amyloidoma" (least common)
- Genetics
  - Sporadic
    - APOE4 allele associated with CAA-related hemorrhage

- Polymorphisms in presenilin-1 gene
  o Hereditary cerebral hemorrhage with amyloidosis
    - Autosomal dominant inheritance
    - Dutch type = mutated amyloid β precursor protein on chromosome 21
    - Other types include British, Flemish, etc.
- Etiology-Pathogenesis-Pathophysiology
  o Amyloidosis = rare systemic disease caused by extracellular deposition of β-amyloid
  o 10-20% localized form, including CNS
  o Can be idiopathic/primary or secondary/reactive (e.g., dialysis-related amyloidosis)
- Epidemiology
  o 1% of all strokes
  o Causes up to 15-20% of primary intracerebral hemorrhage (pICH) in patients > 60y
  o Frequency of CAA in elderly
    - 27-32% of normal elderly (autopsy)
    - 82-88% in patients with Alzheimer disease (AD)
    - Common in Down syndrome

Gross Pathologic or Surgical Features
- Lobar hemorrhage
- Multiple small cortical hemorrhages

Microscopic Features
- Interstitial, vascular/perivascular deposits of amorphous protein
  o Stains with Congo red
  o Birefringent under polarized light
- Microaneurysms
- Fibrinoid necrosis
- Perivascular infiltrates
- Hyaline thickening

Clinical Issues

Presentation
- Spontaneous lobar hemorrhage
- 40% with subacute dementia/overt AD
- 2/3 normotensive; 1/3 HTN

Natural History
- Multiple, recurrent hemorrhages
- Progressive cognitive decline

Treatment & Prognosis
- Evacuate focal hematoma if patient < 75y, no IVH, not parietal
- Low Glasgow Coma scale scores, APOE4 allele adverse prognostic factors

Selected References
1. McCarron MO et al: Cerebral amyloid angiopathy-related hemorrhage. Stroke 30: 1643-6, 1999
2. Good CD et al: Amyloid angiopathy causing widespread miliary haemorrhages within the brain evident on MRI. Neuroradiol 40: 308-11, 1998
3. Chan S et al: Multifocal hypointense cerebral lesions on gradient-echo MR are associated with chronic hypertension. AJNR 17: 1821-7, 1996

Small Vessel Ischemia

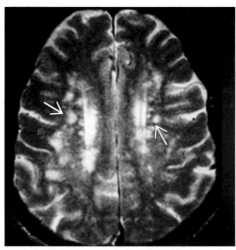

T2WI demonstrates multiple periventricular hyperintensities (arrows) in this 72-year-old-woman.

Key Facts
- Synonyms (common form): Deep white matter ischemia, small vessel ischemic changes, leukoaraiosis
- Synonyms (severe form): Deep white matter infarction, subcortical arteriosclerotic encephalopathy (SAE), Binswanger's disease
- Definition: Ischemic myelin loss in deep white matter and brainstem (common form) to frank subcortical infarction (severe form)
- Classic imaging appearance: T2 hyperintensity in periventricular white matter and central brainstem on MRI
- Ubiquitous and usually asymptomatic in elderly patients; rare cause of dementia (hypertensive white matter vasculopathy or Binswanger's dis.)

Imaging Findings
General Features
- Best imaging clue: T2 hyperintensity in deep white matter and brainstem
CT Findings
- NECT: Ill-defined periventricular hypodensity
- CECT: Same as NECT
MR Findings
- T1WI: Usually normal (severe form: Hypointensity due to cavitation)
- T2WI: Patchy hyperintensity in periventricular region and brainstem
- FLAIR: Hyperintensity parallel to ependyma on sagittal images
- DWI: Normal
Imaging Recommendations
- T2 or FLAIR MRI

Differential Diagnosis
Multiple Sclerosis
- Usually younger patients with recurrent neurologic symptoms
- Hyperintensity perpendicular to ependyma on thin FLAIR sagittal

Small Vessel Ischemia

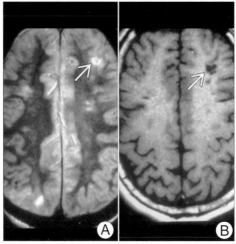

66-year-old man with recent left carotid endarterectomy now with left hemispheric stroke. (A) Proton density weighted image demonstrates subcortical hyperintensity (arrow). (B) T1WI demonstrates CSF intensity, indicating cavitation and infarction (arrow).

Ependymitis Granularis
- T2 hyperintensity parallel to ependyma near frontal horns in patients > 40 years of age
- Represents increased water content in less tightly integrated white matter near frontal horns
- Asymptomatic

Pathology
General
- General Path Comments
  - Medium-sized vessels supplying deep white matter have long parenchymal course
    - More susceptible to drop in blood pressure
    - More susceptible to changes of hypertension and aging than cortical vessels
    - Less able to autoregulate
    - Poor collateralization
  - Perivascular ischemia leading to myelin pallor (common) to infarction (severe)
- Etiology-Pathogenesis
  - Slow occlusion of lenticulostriates, thalamoperforators and brainstem perforators
  - Chronic ischemia leads to death of oligodendroglia and loss of myelin
  - Loss of myelin leads to more hydrophilic environment and T2 increase
  - Slow occlusion results in parallel fibers picking up function, hence lack of symptoms
Gross Pathologic Features
- Pale lesions on a pale background, i.e., poorly seen

Microscopic Features
- Myelin pallor and isomorphic gliosis (common form)
- Frank infarction, i.e., cavitation, axonal loss, and necrosis with surrounding gliosis
  - If subcortical, suggests embolic disease
  - If periventricular, indicates severe form of disease, e.g., SAE

Clinical Issues
Presentation
- Common form: No symptoms
  - No measurable psychometric impairment or focal neurologic symptoms
- Severe form (SAE): Dementia, pseudobulbar palsy, motor signs
- Imaging findings more severe in hypertensives, heavy smokers, and diabetics
Natural History
- Common form: Progressive worsening of MRI with time
- Severe form: Stepwise, cumulative neurologic deficits and dementia
Treatment
- Usually no treatment required
- If hypertensive, antihypertensive medications
Prognosis
- Common form: Excellent
- Severe form: Progressive, stepwise deterioration

Selected References
1. Yetkin FZ et al: Focal hyperintensities in cerebral white matter on MR images of asymptomatic volunteers: correlation with social and medical histories. Am J Roentgenol 161: 855-8, 1993
2. Awad IA et al: Incidental subcortical lesions identified on magnetic resonance imaging in the elderly. I. Correlation with age and cerebral vascular factors. Stroke 17: 1084-9, 1986
3. Awad IA et al: Incidental subcortical lesions identified on magnetic resonance imaging in the elderly. II. Postmortem pathologic correlations. Stroke 17: 1090-7, 1986

Radiation Vasculopathy, CNS

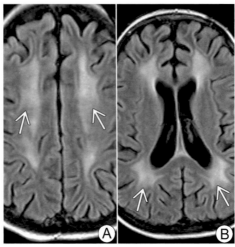

Axial FLAIR images (A, B) demonstrate confluent periventricular hyperintensity (arrows).

Key Facts
- Radiation vasculopathy: Includes edema, arteritis, radiation necrosis, mineralizing microangiopathy, progressive leukoencephalopathy, radiation-induced tumors
- Distinguishing residual/recurrent neoplasm from radiation-induced necrosis difficult using morphology alone
- Functional imaging (PET, SPECT, MRS) may help

Imaging Findings
General Features
- Radiation (XRT) injury varies from mild vasogenic edema to frank necrosis
- Periventricular white matter (WM) especially susceptible

CT Findings
- NECT
  - Confluent low-density WM within radiation port
  - Basal ganglia/gyriform subcortical Ca++ = mineralizing microangiopathy
- CECT
  - Usually does not enhance
  - Necrotizing leukoencephalopathy may have ring-enhancing mass

MR Findings
- Acute: WM hyperintense areas on T2WI/FLAIR (vasogenic edema)
- Chronic
  - **Diffuse WM hyperintensity** on T2WI
    - "Radiation-induced WM changes"
    - More common in older patients
    - Probably reflects preexisting subclinical arteriosclerosis compounded by radiation vasculopathy
  - Radionecrosis of WM
    - Immediate vicinity of tumor/surgical cavity

Radiation Vasculopathy, CNS

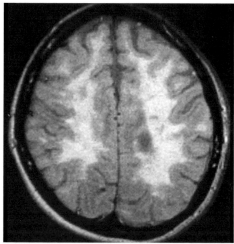

Proton density weighted image in 70-year-old man with whole brain irradiation 2 years previously demonstrates confluent periventricular hyperintensity.

- May cause mass effect, can increase in size
  - Most common: Hypointense rim (T2WI), enhances (resembles recurrent/persistent tumor)
  - Other patterns
    - Multiple lesions remote from tumor site (nodular, linear, curvilinear, "soap bubble" or "Swiss cheese" enhancement)
    - Non-enhancing parenchymal cysts

Other Modality Findings
- MRS: Low N-acetyl aspartate (NAA), Cho normal, lipid elevated
  - Use Cho to distinguish from tumor (Cho elevated in tumor)
- SPECT, PET: Radionecrosis usually hypometabolic (decreased FDG, methionine, ^{201}Tl uptake), reduced rCBV

Imaging Recommendations
- Contrast-enhanced MR, MRS
- PET/SPECT

Differential Diagnosis
Radiation Necrosis vs. Recurrent Neoplasm
- Both often have ring-enhancing mass
- Radionecrosis usually hypometabolic, low rCBV
- Recurrent tumor has high glucose metabolism, Tl uptake with slow washout (NB: False-positives have been reported)

Foreign Body Reaction to Hemostatic Materials
- Granulomatous reaction to gelatin sponge, etc.
- Can mimic tumor recurrence, radiation necrosis
- May require biopsy

Tumor/Edema vs. XRT-Induced Demyelination
- Both have WM hyperintensities
- Both may enhance

Radionecrosis vs. Metastasis, Abscess
- MRS helpful

Radiation Vasculopathy, CNS

Pathology

<u>General</u>
- General Path Comments
  - Variables include: Total radiation dose, radiation field size, radiation fraction size, number/frequency of doses, adjuvant therapy, duration of survival, age of patient
  - Most XRT injury is delayed (at least 1 year)
- Etiology-Pathogenesis
  - Radiation-induced vascular injury
    - Endothelial and basement membrane damage
    - Accelerated atherosclerosis
    - Telangiectasia formation
  - Radiation-induced neurotoxicity
    - Glial and white matter damage (sensitivity of oligodendrocytes >> neurons)
    - Miscellaneous (effects on fibrinolytic system, immune effects)
  - Rare: Radiation-induced tumor (sarcoma, etc.)
- Epidemiology
  - Overall incidence of radionecrosis 5-24%
  - 5% of those radiated for nasopharyngeal SCCa
  - < 18% for external beam RT
  - 25-30% for radiosurgery (gamma knife, X knife)
  - 30-40% for brachytherapy

<u>Gross Pathologic or Surgical Features</u>
- Spectrum from minor abnormalities to gross cavitating WM necrosis

<u>Microscopic Features</u>
- Vascular changes
  - Fibrinoid necrosis of blood vessels
  - Perivascular coagulative necrosis
  - Wall thickening, hyalinization
  - Thrombosis, luminal occlusion
  - Dilated, thin-walled telangiectasias may develop
- White matter changes = focal/diffuse demyelination

Clinical Issues

<u>Presentation</u>
- Highly variable

<u>Natural History</u>
- Radiation-induced necrosis is a dynamic pathophysiological process with several possible clinical outcomes
  - Usually progressive, irreversible
  - Some lesions stabilize, even regress
  - 15-point drop in IQ for external beam (5000 rads)

<u>Treatment & Prognosis</u>
- Biopsy if imaging does not resolve tumor vs. radionecrosis
- Surgery if mass effect, edema

Selected References
1. Chong VF-H et al: Temporal lobe changes following radiation therapy: imaging and proton MRS findings. Eur Radiol 11: 317-24, 2001
2. Kamingo T et al: Radiosurgery-induced microvascular alterations precede necrosis of the brain neuropil. Neurosurg 49: 409-15, 2001
3. Kumar AJ et al: Malignant gliomas: MR imaging spectrum of radiation therapy- and chemotherapy-induced necrosis of the brain after treatment. Radiology 217: 377-84, 2000

Saccular Aneurysm

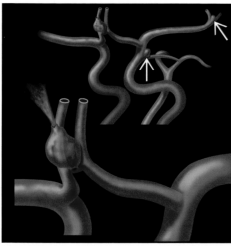

Graphic depiction of the circle of Willis shows a large, lobulated, aCoA aneurysm with rupture into the subarachnoid space. Unruptured aneurysms are also depicted at the MCA and pCoA (arrows).

Key Facts
- Aneurysm formation multifactorial
- Genetics play increasingly recognized role
- Subarachnoid hemorrhage (SAH) most common presentation
- Size most important (but not only) factor in rupture risk

Imaging Findings
General Features
- Best diagnostic sign = round, lobulated or bleb-like outpouching
- Usually arises from vessel bifurcation > lateral wall
- Involves short segment of vessel wall
CT Findings
- Ruptured = high density blood in basal cisterns ("SAH")
- Patent aneurysm
  o Well-delineated, round/lobulated extra-axial mass
  o Slightly hyperdense to brain (may have mural Ca++)
  o Enhances strongly
- Partially/completely thrombosed aneurysm
  o Moderately hyperdense (Ca++ common)
  o Patent lumen enhances
MR Findings
- SAH bright on FLAIR (100%)
  o More sensitive than CT but not as specific due to CSF inflow effects in basal cisterns
- Patent aneurysm (signal varies)
  o 50% have "flow void" (high velocity signal loss)
  o Iso/heterogeneous signal, incomplete delineation
    ▪ Slow/turbulent flow
    ▪ Saturation effects, phase dispersion
- Partially/completely thrombosed aneurysm

Saccular Aneurysm

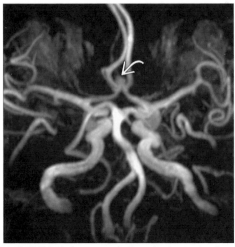

MOTSA MRA of aCoM (anterior communicating artery) aneurysm (curved arrow).

- o Signal depends on age(s) of clot
- o Often hyperintense on T1WI
- o Hypointense on T2WI
- o May be **laminated** with very hypointense rim
- o Patent lumen enhances

Other Modality Findings
- Role of DSA/CTA/MRA
  - o Delineate aneurysm, define neck, detect multiple aneurysms
  - o Identify perforating arteries that may arise from dome
  - o Assess potential for collateral circulation
- Findings
  - o Round/lobulated, focal outpouching, may have apical "tit"
  - o Narrow or broad-based

Imaging Recommendations
- CTA, MRA excellent screening tools for aneurysms > 3-4 mm

Differential Diagnosis

Small Patent Aneurysm
- Vessel loop (use multiple projections)
- Infundibulum (< 3 mm, conical, small pCoA from apex)

Thrombosed Aneurysm
- Hemorrhagic neoplasm, thrombosed vascular malformation

Pathology

General
- Genetics (increasingly recognized role)
  - o Abnormal expression/functional polymorphism of some genes
    - Endoglin, MMP-9
    - Overexpression of other genes encoding extracellular matrix components (e.g., collagen, elastin)
  - o Hereditary, connective tissue disorders
    - Ehlers-Danlos type IV, NF-1

Saccular Aneurysm

- Fibromuscular dysplasia
- Autosomal dominant polycystic kidney disease (10%)
  - o Familial intracranial aneurysms (no known heritable disorder)
    - Occur in "clusters" (two first-order relatives)
    - 10% prevalence (vs. 1-2% autopsy prevalence)
    - Significantly younger patients
    - Up to 20% of all acute SAH
- Etiology-Pathogenesis-Pathophysiology
  - o Flow-related "bioengineering fatigue" in vessel wall
  - o Abnormal vascular hemodynamics
    - Arises at areas of high biomechanical stress
    - Abnormal slipstream vectors
    - Higher/disturbed flow, increased pulsatility
- Epidemiology
  - o From 1.22/100,000 person-yr (age 0-34) to 44.47/100,000 person-yr (age 65-74)
    - Women > men (especially with multiple aneurysms)
  - o Rare in children
    - 1-2% of all aneurysms
    - Different location (ICA bifurcation, M2 MCA)
  - o 20% multiple

Gross Pathologic or Surgical Features
- Round/lobulated sac, thin or thick wall, +/- SAH

Microscopic Features
- Disrupted/absent internal elastic lamina
- Muscle layer absent
- May have "tit" of fragile adventitia

Clinical Issues

Presentation
- Intracranial hemorrhage 60-85%
  - o Headache (often "thunderclap")
- Other: "Migraine," cranial neuropathy, TIA, seizure

Natural History (Rupture Risk)
- Size (small if < 10 mm, high if > 25 mm)
- Shape (multilobed, "tit", aspect ratio > 1.6)
- "Perianeurysmal environment" (contact with other structures)?
- Other (hypertension, female gender, smoking)

Selected References
1.   Proust F et al: Pediatric cerebral aneurysms. J Neurosurg 94: 733-9, 2001
2.   White PM et al: Intracranial aneurysms: CTA and MRA for detection. Radiol 219: 739-49, 2001
3.   Menghini W et al: Clinical manifestations and survival rates among patients with saccular intracranial aneurysms. Neurosurg 49: 251-8, 2001

Fusiform Aneurysm (FA)

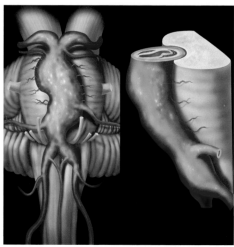

Graphic depicts atherosclerotic fusiform aneurysm of the vertebrobasilar system.

Key Facts
- Fusiform aneurysm (FA) less common than saccular aneurysm
- FAs involve long, nonbranching vessel segments
- Can be acute (dissecting aneurysm) or chronic (ASVD, nonatherosclerotic vasculopathy)

Imaging Findings
General Features
- Best diagnostic sign = long segment fusiform or ovoid arterial dilatation
CT Findings
- NECT: Hyperdense; Ca++ common
- CECT: Lumen enhances strongly, intramural clot does not
MR Findings
- Ectatic vessel +/- more focal aneurysmal outpouching
- Mixed signal intensity common, varies with
  - Flow velocity, direction, turbulence
    - Slow flow seen as high signal deep into imaged sections
  - Presence, age of mural hematoma
    - Often hyperintense on T1WI, hypointense rim on T2WI
    - Clot may be laminated (layers of organized thrombus at different stages of evolution)
- Residual lumen enhances strongly
Other Modality Findings
- MRA
  - Precontrast 3D-TOF may be inadequate because of
    - Flow saturation effects
    - Intravoxel phase dispersion
  - Giant FA usually requires dynamic contrast-enhanced sequences for accurate delineation
- DSA/CTA
  - Exaggerated arterial ectasia(s)
  - More focal fusiform or even saccular enlargement may occur

54

Fusiform Aneurysm (FA)

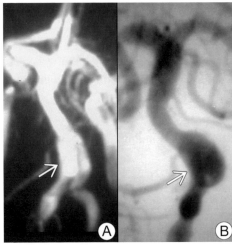

Fusiform aneurysm of basilar artery (arrows) in sickle cell patient. (A) MOTSA MRA. (B) DSA.

o Can be solitary or multifocal

Differential Diagnosis
Vertebrobasilar Dolichoectasia
• Older patient
• Changes of ASVD in other vessels
• Ectasia often extends into branches
Giant Serpentine Aneurysm
• Large, partially thrombosed mass
• Distal branches arise from aneurysm dome
• Lacks definable neck
• May be indistinguishable from FA
Nonatherosclerotic Fusiform Vasculopathy
• Younger patient
• History of inherited vasculopathy, immune disorder

Pathology
General
• FAs can be atherosclerotic, nonatherosclerotic
• Nonatherosclerotic fusiform and dissecting aneurysms
  o Type 1 = typical dissecting aneurysm
  o Type 2 = segmental ectasias
  o Type 3 = dolichoectatic dissecting aneurysms
  o Type 4 = atypically located saccular aneurysm (i.e., lateral wall, unrelated to branching zones)
• Genetics
  o Marfan syndrome: Mutation of fibrillin genes (FBN1)
• Etiology-Pathogenesis
  o Atherosclerosis usual cause of basilar FA in older adults
    ▪ Lipid deposition is initial step
    ▪ Internal elastic lamina (IEL): Muscle layers become disrupted

Fusiform Aneurysm (FA)

- Enhanced susceptibility to hemodynamic stress
  o Nonatherosclerotic fusiform aneurysms
    - IEL fragmentation is initial step
    - Immune deficiency (e.g., HIV)
    - Viral, other infectious agents (e.g., Varicella)
    - Collagen vascular disorders (e.g., SLE)
    - Sickle cell anemia

Gross Pathologic or Surgical Features
- Focally dilated fusiform arterial ectasia(s)
- +/- ASVD

Microscopic Features
- Type 1 = widespread disruption of the IEL, no intimal thickening
- Type 2 = extended and/or fragmented IEL with intimal thickening
- Type 3 = IEL fragmentation, multiple dissections of thickened intima, organized thrombus
- Type 4 = absent IEL, muscular layer

Clinical Issues
Presentation
- Headache, subarachnoid hemorrhage
- TIA, cranial neuropathy

Natural History
- Type 1: Rebleed common
- Type 2: Benign clinical course
- Type 3: Slow but progressive enlargement
- Type 4: Rerupture risk high

Treatment & Prognosis
- Often combined surgical, endovascular
- 80% of giant "unclippable" aneurysms dead/disabled at 5 years

Selected References
1. Jager HR et al: Contrast-enhanced MR angiography of intracranial giant aneurysms. AJNR 21: 1900-7, 2000
2. Nakatomi H et al: Clinicopathological study of intracranial fusiform and dolichoectatic aneurysms. Stroke 31: 896-900, 2000
3. Mizutani T et al: Proposed classification of nonatherosclerotic cerebral fusiform and dissecting aneurysms. Neurosurg 45: 253-60, 1999

Sagittal Sinus Thrombosis

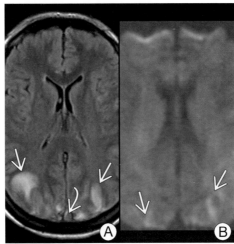

(A) FLAIR axial image demonstrates bilateral parasagittal parietal hyperintensities (arrows) and no flow void in the expected position of superior sagittal sinus (curved arrow) due to thrombosis. (B) Diffusion image demonstrates ischemia (arrows), i.e., venous infarcts.

Key Facts
- 1% of acute strokes
- Clinical diagnosis often elusive
- Early imaging findings may be subtle, often overlooked

Imaging Findings
General Features
- Thrombus in dural sinus, vein(s)
- Parenchymal edema, petechial hemorrhages
- Best diagnostic sign = "empty delta" on CECT, contrast-enhanced MR

CT Findings
- NECT
  - Hyperdense dural sinus > cortical vein ("cord sign")
  - +/- Parenchymal abnormality
    - Cortical/subcortical petechial hemorrhages, edema
    - If internal cerebral veins (ICVs) occlude, thalami/basal ganglia are hypodense
- CECT
  - "Empty delta" sign (enhancing dura surrounds nonenhancing thrombus) in 25-30% of cases
  - "Shaggy," irregular veins (collateral channels)

MR Findings
- Signal varies with age of clot
  - Acute
    - Absent "flow void"
    - Clot isointense on T1WI, hypointense on T2WI
  - Subacute: Hyperintense on unenhanced T1-, T2WI
- Venous infarct (50% of cases)
  - Gyral swelling, sulcal effacement
    - Hyperintense (T2WI, FLAIR)

Sagittal Sinus Thrombosis

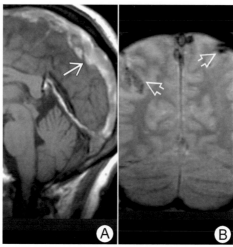

*(A) Sagittal T1WI demonstrates subacute thrombus (methemoglobin) in superior sagittal sinus (arrow). (B) Coronal T2*WI demonstrates bilateral, parasagittal foci of hypointensity (open arrows) consistent with intracellular deoxy- or met-hemoglobin, i.e., acute or early subacute hemorrhage (venous infarcts).*

- Petechial hemorrhage (cortical/subcortical)
  - Patchy enhancement

Other Modality Findings
- MRV/CTV
  - Loss of vascular flow signal
  - "Frayed" or "shaggy" appearance of venous sinus
  - Abnormal collateral channels (e.g., enlarged medullary veins)
  - Do phase contrast MRV – TOF MRV is falsely negative if clot subacute
- DWI/ADC imaging findings variable, heterogeneous
  - < 3 weeks: DWI positive
  - > 3 weeks: DWI normal
- SPECT/PET: Decreased rCBF

Imaging Recommendations
- NECT, CECT scans +/- CTV
- If CT scan negative, MRI with MRV
- If MRV equivocal, DSA

Differential Diagnosis

Normal
- Blood in vessels normally slightly hyperdense on NECT scans

Anatomic Variant
- Congenital hypoplastic/absent transverse sinus
- "High-splitting" tentorium

"Giant" Arachnoid Granulation
- Round/ovoid filling defect (clot is long, linear)
- CSF density/signal intensity

False "Empty Delta" Sign
- SDH, SDE

Sagittal Sinus Thrombosis

Neoplasm
- Venous infarct can enhance, mimic neoplasm

Pathology
General
- Genetics (inherited predisposing conditions)
  - Resistance to activated protein C (typically due to factor V Leiden mutation) = most common cause of sporadic cerebral vascular thrombosis (CVT)
  - Protein S deficiency
  - Prothrombin (factor II) gene mutation (G20210A)
- Etiology-Pathogenesis-Pathophysiology
  - Wide spectrum of causes (> 100 identified)
    - Trauma, infection, inflammation
    - Pregnancy, oral contraceptives
    - Metabolic (dehydration, thyrotoxicosis, cirrhosis, etc.)
    - Hematological (coagulopathy)
    - Collagen-vascular disorders (e.g., APLA syndrome)
    - Vasculitis (e.g., Behcet)
  - Most common pattern: Thrombus initially forms in dural sinus
    - Clot propagates into cortical veins
    - Venous drainage obstructed, venous pressure elevated
    - BBB breakdown with vasogenic edema, hemorrhage
    - Venous infarct with cytotoxic edema ensues
- Epidemiology: 1% of acute strokes
Gross Pathologic or Surgical Features
- Sinus occluded, distended by acute clot
- Thrombus in adjacent cortical veins
- Adjacent cortex edematous, usually with petechial hemorrhage
Staging or Grading Criteria
- Venous ischemia
  - Type 1: No abnormality
  - Type 2: High signal on T2WI/FLAIR; no enhancement
  - Type 3: High signal on T2WI/FLAIR; enhancement present
  - Type 4: Hemorrhage or venous infarction

Clinical Issues
Presentation
- Extremely variable (from asymptomatic to coma, death)
- Common: Headache, nausea, vomiting +/- neurologic deficit
Natural History
- Up to 50% of cases progress to venous infarction
- Potentially fatal
Treatment & Prognosis
- Heparin +/- rtPA
- Endovascular thrombolysis

Selected References
1. Liang L et al: Evaluation of the intracranial dural sinuses with a 3D contrast-enhanced MP-RAGE sequence. AJNR 22: 481-92, 2001
2. Kawaguchi T et al: Classification of venous ischemia with MRI. J Clin Neurosci 8 (suppl 1): 82-8, 2001
3. Provenzale JM et al: Dural sinus thrombosis: Findings on CT and MR imaging and diagnostic pitfalls. AJR 170: 777-83, 1998

Hypertensive Encephalopathy

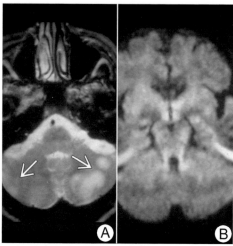

11-year-old girl with acute lymphocytic leukemia and acute "stroke". (A) T2WI demonstrates bilateral cerebellar hyperintensities consistent with ischemic stroke (arrows). (B) Diffusion image through same level as (A) is normal.

Key Facts
- Synonyms: Posterior reversible encephalopathy syndrome (PRES), reversible posterior leukoencephalopathy syndrome
- Definition: Extravasation of serum across a temporary defect in the blood brain barrier due to a high pressure gradient
- Classic imaging appearance: Posterior symmetric bilateral parasagittal hyperintensities on T2W MRI (with normal diffusion imaging) which returns to normal if hypertension controlled

Imaging Findings
General Features
- Best imaging clue: Posterior parasagittal hyperintensities on T2W MRI with normal diffusion imaging
CT Findings
- NECT: Posterior parasagittal hypodensities
- CECT: Same as NECT unless infarction in which case gyral enhancement
MR Findings
- T1WI: Subtle posterior parasagittal hypointensities
- T2WI and FLAIR: Bilateral parasagittal hyperintensities involving the posterior frontal, parietal, and occipital lobes as well as the cerebellum and occasionally the basal ganglia and brainstem
- Diffusion imaging: Early – normal; if hypertension (HTN) not treated, could be positive for infarction
Imaging Recommendations
- T2W MRI or FLAIR with diffusion imaging

Differential Diagnosis
Superior Sagittal Sinus (SSS) Thrombosis
- Can also give posterior parasagittal hyperintensities on T2WI
- Diffusion imaging initially positive, becoming normal after 3 weeks

Hypertensive Encephalopathy

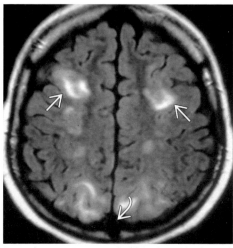

Axial FLAIR image demonstrates parasagittal hyperintensities (arrows) in a patient with patent SSS (curved arrow) and negative diffusion study.

- Thrombus seen in SSS

<u>Acute Disseminated Encephalomyelitis (ADEM)</u>
- Can give bilateral white matter hyperintensities on T2WI
- May be positive on diffusion imaging due to acute demyelination

Pathology
<u>General</u>
- General Path Comments
  - Edema of the cortical and subcortical posterior parietal and occipital lobes with petechial microhemorrhages
- Anatomy
  - Posterior > anterior circulation due to decreased sympathetic enervation posteriorly and decreased autoregulation of arteriolar precapillary vasomotor tone
- Etiology-Pathogenesis: Temporary, reversible "leak" in blood brain barrier
  - Under large pressure gradient due to severe hypertension; can be
    - Acute due to rise in systemic hypertension
    - Chronic from essential or from chronic HTN due to renal or collagen vascular disease
  - Common causes: Eclampsia-preeclampsia syndrome
  - Less common causes: Thrombotic thrombocytopenic purpura, hemolytic-uremic syndrome, cyclosporine toxicity
  - Proposed mechanism
    - Resulting transudate called "reversible vasogenic edema"
    - When autoregulatory limits are exceeded, the cerebral arteriole passively overdistends
    - Results in distraction of the tight junctions between endothelial cells
    - Extravasation of fluid and proteins across an altered blood-brain barrier

Hypertensive Encephalopathy

- Results in "reversible" vasogenic edema which migrates from the tightly integrated gray matter to the white matter

Microscopic Features
- Subcortical vasogenic edema with petechial microhemorrhages
- Fibrinoid necrosis of arteriolar walls
- Infarction not found unless treatment delayed

Clinical Issues
Presentation
- Headaches, nausea, vomiting, seizures, visual disturbances, altered consciousness, coma
- Most common cause: Toxemia of pregnancy

Natural History
- If HTN not treated, cerebral infarction or intracranial hemorrhage will result

Treatment
- Antihypertensives
- Magnesium sulfate for eclampsia, preeclampsia

Prognosis
- Good if hypertension controlled
- Poor if hypertension not controlled

Selected References
1. Provenzale JM et al: Quantitative assessment of diffusion abnormalities in posterior reversible encephalopathy syndrome. AJNR 22: 1455-61, 2001
2. Casey SO et al: "Posterior reversible encephalopathy syndrome: Utility of fluid-attenuated inversion recovery MR imaging in the detection of cortical and subcortical lesions". AJNR 21: 1199-206, 2000
3. Cooney MJ et al: Hypertensive encephalopathy: Complication in children treated for myeloproliferative fisorders-report of three cases. Radiology 214: 711-6, 2000

Cavernous Sinus Thrombosis

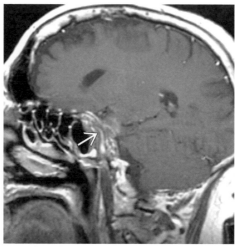

Sagittal contrast-enhanced T1WI in a patient with septic cavernous sinus thrombosis shows narrowing and slow flow in the right internal carotid artery (arrow). (Courtesy Anne G Osborn MD)

Key Facts
- Synonym: CST
- Definition: Thrombosis of the cavernous sinus (CS) or its tributaries
- Classic imaging appearance
  - CT/MR: Enlarged CS and superior ophthalmic vein (SOV) with post-contrast filling defects
- Other key facts
  - May occur in association with a carotid cavernous fistula (CCF) (aseptic, spontaneous)
  - Septic thrombophlebitis rare in antibiotic era
  - Fever and meningitis signal septic thrombophlebitis
  - CS = Fourth most common occluded dural sinus (after superior sagittal, transverse and sigmoid)

Imaging Findings
General Features
- Best imaging clue
  - Enlarged CS and SOV with filling defects post enhancement
CT Findings
- NECT
  - CS may have convex walls
  - CS may be high density, occasionally contain air
  - Enlarged SOV, proptosis with periorbital soft tissue swelling
  - Look for associated findings (e.g., sinusitis)
- CECT
  - May show filling defects
MR Findings
- Absence of flow voids on routine MR
- Low signal intensity acute clot in CS, SOV on T2WI
- Multiple filling defects seen in sinus on T1WI + Gd

Cavernous Sinus Thrombosis

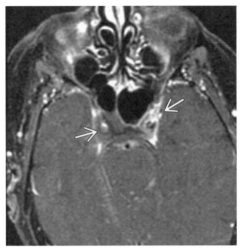

Same case as previous page. Axial post-contrast enhanced T1WI shows non-enhancing filling defects within the enhancing thrombosed cavernous sinus (arrows). Note slight convenxity of CS walls. (Courtesy Anne G Osborn MD)

<u>MRA/CTA Findings</u>
- Flow sensitive (TOF) sequences reveal thrombosis of cavernous veins
- May see narrowing/thrombosis of cavernous ICA with thrombophlebitis

<u>Other Modality Findings</u>
- DSA may delineate presence of CCF, thrombosis (usually unnecessary unless pre-embolization)

<u>Imaging Recommendations</u>
- Contrast enhanced MR or CT

Differential Diagnosis

<u>Carotid Cavernous Fistula</u>
- Exophthalmos with tortuosity and dilatation of superior ophthalmic veins
- Rupture of ICA (direct) or its dural branches (indirect) results in sudden shunting of arterial blood into the cavernous sinus
- MRA/CTA reveals high flow fistula with venous hypertension
- May cause "spontaneous" CST

<u>Tolosa-Hunt Syndrome</u>
- Idiopathic inflammatory condition of cavernous sinus, superior orbital fissure and orbital apex
- Painful ophthalmoplegia (CN III, IV, VI) and V1 hypesthesia
- Steroid responsive

Pathology

<u>General</u>
- Etiology-Pathogenesis
  - "Spontaneous" (associated with CCF)
  - Septic (secondary to infection of paranasal sinuses and/or orbit)

Cavernous Sinus Thrombosis

Clinical Issues

Presentation

- When associated with CCF, CST presents as sudden onset or exacerbation of proptosis, chemosis and periorbital soft-tissue swelling
- Septic CST associated with fever and signs of meningeal irritation
- May be associated with CS cranial neuropathies and CVA due to narrowing of ICA
- Potentially lethal if not treated

Treatment

- Directed to predisposing cause
  - o Paranasal sinus infection
    - Functional endoscopy
    - Antibiotics
  - o CCF
    - Endovascular closure of fistula

Prognosis

- Excellent with early diagnosis, appropriate treatment
- CCF 90% cure after embolization

Selected References
1. Ellie E et al: CT and high-field MRI in septic thrombosis of the cavernous sinuses. Neuroradiology 34(1): 22-4, 1992
2. Ahmadi J et al: CT observations pertinent to septic cavernous sinus thrombosis. AJNR 6(5): 755-8, 1985
3. Clifford-Jones RE et al: Cavernous sinus thrombosis. J Neurol Neurosurg Psychiatry 45(12): 1092-7, 1982

Carotid Pseudoaneurysm, Intracranial

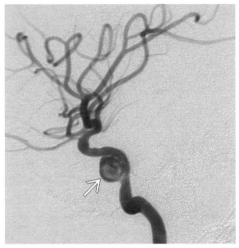

Left internal carotid angiogram, arterial phase, lateral view, in a 15-year-old male with a comminuted skull base fracture (not shown). A pseudoaneurysm of the cavernous internal carotid artery (ICA) is present (arrow).

Key Facts
- Synonym: False aneurysm
- Definition: Cavitated, organized thrombus without normal layers of vessel wall
- Classic imaging appearance: Irregular, contrast-filled paravascular mass
- Most common cause = trauma
- Intracranial dissections, dissecting aneurysms, and pseudoaneurysms are rare but important causes of subarachnoid hemorrhage (SAH)
- High mortality, morbidity, so early diagnosis and treatment essential

Imaging Findings
General Features
- Best imaging clue: Irregular/lobulated dilatation of cerebral artery
- Pseudoaneurysms usually involve cavernous internal carotid artery (ICA) or distal medial cerebral artery (MCA)/anterior cerebral artery (ACA) at nonbranching points

CT Findings
- NECT
  - Iso/hyperdense paravascular mass
    - Corpus callosum is common site
  - +/- Identifiable fracture
    - Most common location = skull base
    - Second most common = calvarium
  - +/- SAH
- CECT: False lumen enhances strongly

MR Findings
- T1WI
  - Signal varies with age of hematoma
  - Usually iso-/hyperintense
- T2WI: Mixed signal common

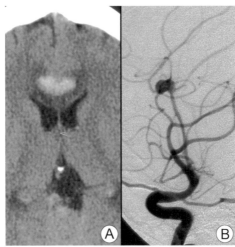

(A) NECT scan in a patient with closed head injury 5 days after trauma shows a focal hematoma near the corpus callosum genu. (B) DSA of the internal carotid artery shows a lobulated distal ACA aneurysm. Surgery disclosed traumatic pseudoaneurysm.

- FLAIR: May show SAH
- GRE: May show other injuries (e.g., diffuse axonal injury (DAI), contusions)
- Contrast-enhanced T1WI: If patent, false lumen enhances strongly

Other Modality Findings
- DSA/CTA
  - Pseudoaneurysms typically fill late, empty slowly
  - Most do not have a definable "neck"
- MRA caution: Subacute hematomas have short T1, may be difficult to distinguish simple clot from pseudoaneurysm unless contrast given

Imaging Recommendations
- Screening MR + contrast-enhanced MRA
- DSA

Differential Diagnosis

Saccular ("True") Aneurysm
- Usually involves circle of Willis or major vessel bifurcation
- Usually not associated with trauma, infection

Dissecting Aneurysm
- Intracranial dissections are rare
- Vertebral artery = most common site
- Supraclinoid ICA, horizontal MCA less commonly involved

Pathology

General
- General Path Comments
  - Paravascular hematoma forms, organizes, cavitates and communicates with true lumen of parent vessel

Carotid Pseudoaneurysm, Intracranial

- o Most involve distal cortical branches (MCA > ACA) or ICA (usually cavernous segment)
- Etiology-Pathogenesis
  - o Damage to all layers of vessel wall
  - o Most intracranial pseudoaneurysms occur in setting of significant craniocerebral trauma
    - Direct (penetrating) injury (stab or gunshot wound)
    - Indirect (e.g., closed head injury with artery impacting against bone or dura)
    - May occur with or without associated skull fracture
  - o Less common causes
    - Infection ("mycotic" pseudoaneurysm)
    - Neoplasm ("oncotic" pseudoaneurysm)
- Epidemiology
  - o Pseudoaneurysms account for < 1% of all intracranial aneurysms

Gross Pathologic or Surgical Features
- Organized paravascular hematoma

Microscopic Features
- Wall of pseudoaneurysm consists of organized thrombus
- No intima, internal elastic lamina, or media
- May be contained by adventitia

Clinical Issues

Presentation
- 50% have devastating hemorrhage
  - o Can be subarachnoid, subdural, intraparenchymal or combination
  - o Can present with massive epistaxis (petrous/cavernous ICA injury, usually with BOS fracture)
- Cranial nerve palsy from hematoma, herniation

Natural History
- Can have delayed presentation (mean = 2-3 weeks after trauma)
- Can remain asymptomatic for years
- Cavernous ICA pseudoaneurysm can rupture, form C-C fistula

Treatment
- Surgical
- Endovascular (coil, trapping)

Prognosis
- High morbidity, mortality with rupture
- Cerebral ischemia if parent vessel occludes

Selected References
1. Guyot LL et al: Vascular injury in neurotrauma. Neurol Res 23: 291-6, 2001
2. Uzan M et al: Traumatic intracranial carotid tree aneurysms. Neurosurg 43: 1314-22, 1998
3. Holmes B et al: Traumatic intracranial aneurysms: A contemporary review. J Trauma 35: 855-60, 1993

Moya-Moya

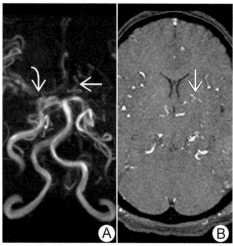

14-year-old sickle cell patient with bilateral distal ICA stenoses, L > R. (A) MRA shows stenosis of R MCA proximally (curved arrow). L MCA is occluded with enlarged lenticulostriate collaterals (arrow). (B) Source image from (A) shows punctate moya-moya collaterals (arrow).

Key Facts
- Synonym: Idiopathic progressive arteriopathy of childhood
- Definition: Progressive narrowing of distal ICA and proximal circle of Willis (COW) vessels with secondary collateralization
- Classic imaging appearance: Multiple punctate dots in basal ganglia
  - Lenticulostriate collaterals
  - "Puff of smoke" ("moya-moya" in Japanese) on angiography
  - Initially described in Japanese children (still most common)
- Increased incidence of stroke
  - Intracranial hemorrhage in adults
  - Sudden hemiplegia in childhood or adolescence

Imaging Findings
General Features
- Best imaging clue: Abnormal netlike vessels at base of brain on A/G
CT Findings
- NECT (children): 50-60% show atrophy usually in anterior circulation
- NECT (adults): Intracranial hemorrhage
- CECT (children): Enhancing dots in basal ganglia (big lenticulostriates)
MR Findings (Children)
- T1WI: Multiple dark dots in basal ganglia
  - Gadolinium turns dots bright, confirming vascular etiology
- T2WI: High signal from small vessel infarcts in cortex and white matter
- MRA: Narrowing of distal ICA and proximal COW vessels
  - Source images demonstrate punctate vessels in basal ganglia
  - Caveat: Anemia and geometry of siphon increase turbulence which can simulate stenosis on bright blood techniques; use black blood MRA
- Diffusion: Positive in acute stroke setting

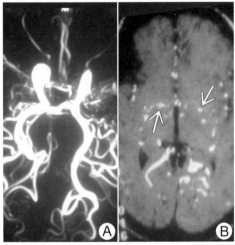

7-year-old girl with sickle cell anemia and severe moya-moya. (A) 3DTOF MRA shows bilateral occlusion of the MCAs. (B) Source images from (A) demonstrate punctate lenticulostriate collaterals (arrows), i.e., moya-moya.

MR Findings (Adults)
- Intracranial (often intraventricular) hemorrhage

Other Modality Findings
- Catheter angiography: Narrowing of proximal COW and ICA (earliest)
  - Lenticulostriate and thalamoperforator collaterals (intermediate)
  - Transdural and transosseous EC-IC collaterals (late disease)
    - Better visualized by catheter angio than MRA

Imaging Recommendations
- MRI of brain for prior stroke (use FLAIR) or hemorrhage (use GRE)
- 3D TOF MRA through COW
  - If normal, stop
  - If supraclinoid carotid stenosis suspected, do black blood MRA
  - If stenosis confirmed, catheter angio to better depict EC-IC collaterals

Differential Diagnosis

Dissection
- Traumatic, spontaneous, underlying vasculopathy

Catheter Spasm
- Reversible stenosis above catheter tip

Vasospasm
- SAH, trauma, infection

Tumor Encasement
- Pituitary adenoma, craniopharyngioma, nasopharyngeal squamous cell carcinoma

Pathology

General
- General Path Comments
  - Results from any slowly progressive intracranial vascular occlusive disorder

Moya-Moya

- Etiology-Pathogenesis: Idiopathic, probably multiple etiologies
  - Usually acquired; 7% familial (in Japan)
  - Atherosclerosis, radiation angiopathy, TB meningitis, leptospirosis, connective tissue disease
  - Sickle cell disease, neurofibromatosis
  - Skull base inflammation, e.g., tonsillitis and otitis media
- Epidemiology
  - Most often in Japanese or black children with sickle cell

Gross Pathologic or Surgical Features
- Increased perforating (early) and EC-IC (late) collaterals in atrophic brain
- Intracranial hemorrhage (adults)
- Increased saccular aneurysms, espicially, basilar (adults)

Microscopic Features
- Intimal thickening
- Excessive infolding and thickening of internal elastic lamina
- Increased periventricular pseudoaneurysms (cause of hemorrhage)

Staging Criteria (After Susuki)
- Stage I: Narrowing of ICA bifurcation
- Stage II: ACA, MCA, PCA dilated
- Stage III: Maximal moya-moya at base of brain; small ACA and MCA
- Stage IV: Fewer moya-moya vessels; small PCA
- Stage V: Further reduction in moya-moya; absent ACA, MCA, PCA
- Stage VI: Extensive pial collaterals from external carotid branches

Clinical Issues

Presentation
- In childhood: TIAs and strokes
- In adulthood: SAH and intraventricular hemorrhage

Natural History
- Steadily progressive narrowing, collateralization and increasing ischemic or hemorrhagic strokes

Treatment
- Perivascular sympathectomy or superior cervical ganglionectomy

Prognosis
- Depends on etiology and age and stage at diagnosis

Selected References
1. Brown WD et al: Moyamoya disease: MR findings. J Comput Assist Tomogr 13(4): 720, 1989
2. Yonekawa Y et al: Moyamoya disease: Diagnosis, treatment, and recent achievement. In Barnett HJM, ed: Stroke: Pathophysiology, diagnosis and management, Vol 2, London, Churchill Livingston, 1986
3. Suzuki J et al: Moyamoya disease-a review. Stroke 14: 104-9, 1983

Vasculitis, Intracranial

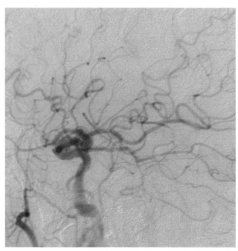

Left common carotid angiogram, arterial phase, lateral view, shows multifocal areas of stenosis and dilatation. Primary arteritis of the central nervous system. (Courtesy Anne G Osborn MD)

Key Facts
- Synonym: Inflammatory vasculopathy, angiitis
- Definition: Heterogeneous group of CNS disorders characterized by inflammation and necrosis of blood vessel walls
- Classic imaging appearance: Variety of angiographic appearances depending on etiology including vascular irregularities, stenoses, aneurysms and occlusions
- Other key facts
  - Infectious and noninfectious etiologies
  - Can be primary intracranial or secondary to a systemic disease

Imaging Findings
General Features
- Best imaging clue: Irregularities, stenoses and vascular occlusions in a pattern or population atypical for atherosclerotic disease
- Imaging workup can be normal; need clinical/laboratory correlation
CT Findings
- Can be normal
- Multifocal low density areas in basal ganglia, subcortical white matter
MR Findings
- Multifocal hyperintensities on T2WI; GRE may show hemorrhage
- Patchy enhancement
DSA
- Alternating stenosis, dilatation primarily involving 2nd, 3rd order branches
- Less common: Long segment stenoses, pseudoaneurysms
CTA/MRA
- Useful screening; spatial resolution may be insufficient for subtle disease
Imaging Recommendations
- MR + MRA
- Conventional angiography if lab studies +, MR/MRA negative

Vasculitis, Intracranial

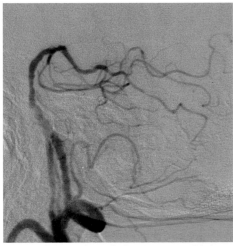

Same case as previous page. Left vertebral angiogram, arterial phase, lateral view, shows beaded appearance of the vertebral and basilar arteries as well as multifocal alternating stenoses and dilatations of smaller branches. (Courtesy Anne G Osborn MD)

Differential Diagnosis

Arterial Vasospasm
- Temporal relationship to subarachnoid hemorrhage (SAH)
- Involves proximal vasculature
- Basilar meningitis may mimic SAH

Intracranial ASVD
- Advanced patient age
- Typical distribution (carotid siphon, proximal intracranial vessels

Pathology

Etiologies: Infectious and Noninfectious Etiologies
- Bacterial meningitis
  - Common in children
  - H. Influenzae most common organism
  - Infarction due to vascular involvement seen in 25%
- Tuberculous meningitis
  - Vessels at the skull base most commonly involved, i.e., supraclinoid ICA and M1 producing occlusions and stenoses
- Mycotic arteritis (aspergillus, cocci, etc)
  - Actinomyces may invade vessel walls leading to hemorrhage
  - Narrowing of the basal cerebral or cortical vessels on angiography
- Viral arteritis
  - Herpes simplex most common in North America
  - HIV-associated vasculitis increasing, especially in children
- Syphilis arteritis
  - Two forms: Syphilitic meningitis and gummatous vasculitis
  - Diffuse vasculitis involves cortical arteries and veins
  - Gummatous vasculitis usually affects proximal MCA branches
- Polyarteritis nodosa

Vasculitis, Intracranial

- o Most common systemic vasculitis to involve the CNS (though late)
- o CNS involvement late
- o Microaneurysms due to necrosis of the internal elastic lamina in 75%
- Cell mediated arteritides
  - o Giant cell arteritis (granulomatous infiltration of the arterial walls)
  - o Takayasu's (primarily involves aorta, great vessels, branches)
  - o Temporal arteritis (systemic; involves temporal, other extracranial arteries)
- Granulomatous angiitis
  - o Primary angiitis isolated to the CNS (idiopathic)
    - ▪ Manifest as multiple intracranial stenoses
  - o Wegener's
    - ▪ Chronic systemic arteritis involving lungs, kidneys and sinuses
    - ▪ CNS involved in 15-30% due to direct invasion from nose/sinuses
    - ▪ May cause intracerebral and meningeal granulomas or vasculitis
  - o Sarcoid (CNS involvement in 3-5% of cases)
    - ▪ Meningitis, vasculitis involving vessels at the base of the brain
    - ▪ Can extend along perivascular spaces, involve penetrating arteries
- Collagen vascular disease (SLE, rheumatoid, scleroderma)
  - o SLE: Most common to involve the CNS
  - o Vasculitis relatively uncommon (variable findings; small vessel irregularities/stenoses/occlusions up to fusiform aneurysms)
  - o CVA seen in 50% due to cardiac disease or coagulopathy
- Drug abuse vasculitis
  - o Drug can injure vessels directly or secondarily (usually hypersensitivity to contaminants)
  - o Associated with both legitimate and illegal "street" drugs including amphetamines, cocaine, heroin, and phenylpropanolmine and ergots
- Radiation
  - o Acute arteritis produces transient white matter edema
  - o Chronic changes more severe with vessel obliteration and brain necrosis, leukomalacia, calcifying microangiopathy and atrophy
  - o Effects compounded with concomitant chemotherapy

Microscopic Features
- Inflammation and necrosis of blood vessel walls

Clinical Issues
Presentation
- Clinical presentation as stroke related to manifestations of vascular involvement (stenosis, occlusion, aneurysm)

Selected References
1. Calabrese LH et al: Diagnostic strategies in vasculitis affecting the central nervous system. Cleve Clin J Med 69 Suppl 2: SII105-8, 2002
2. Wasserman BA et al: Reliability of normal findings on MR imaging for excluding the diagnosis of vasculitis of the central nervous system. AJR 177(2): 455-9, 2001
3. Harris KG et al: Diagnosing intracranial vasculitis: The roles of MR and angiography. AJNR 15(2): 17-30, 1994

Dural AV Shunts, Brain

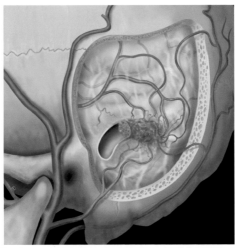

Graphic with cutaway of transverse sinus depicts a dural AV shunts. The sinus is thrombosed and numerous "crack-like" vessels are present in the sinus wall. Supply is from dural branches of both ECA and ICA.

Key Facts
- Dural AV shunts (dAVSs) also known as dural arteriovenous fistulae (dAVFs)
- Cluster of numerous "micro" AV shunts inside dural sinus wall
- Most are acquired, express active angiogenesis
- Clinical manifestations vary with location, presence of venous hypertension

Imaging Findings
General Features
- Adult-type dAVS
  - Best diagnostic sign = network of tiny "crack-like" vessels in thrombosed dural sinus
- Infantile dAVS (rare)
  - Best diagnostic sign = multiple high-flow shunts involving different dural sinuses
CT Findings
- NECT: Often normal
- CECT
  - May be normal with small shunts
  - +/- Serpentine feeders, enlarged dural sinus
  - Enlarged superior ophthalmic vein (with carotid cavernous fistula)
  - 3D / CTA may be useful in static depiction of angioarchitecture
MR Findings
- May be normal
- Thrombosed transverse/sigmoid sinus (TS/SS) contains numerous flow voids from "micro" fistulae ("crack-like" vessels)
Other Modality Findings
- DSA
  - Most common = TS or SS dAVS
    - Dural sinus often thrombosed

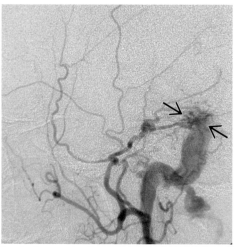

53-year-old female who presents with pulsatile tinnitus (right external carotid injection, lateral view). There is a fistulous connection between the middle meningeal artery and the sigmoid-transverse junction (arrows). (Courtesy Peter Schloesser MD)

- Flow reversal in dural sinus/cortical correlates with progressive symptoms, risk of hemorrhage
- Tortuous engorged pial veins ("pseudophlebitic pattern") with venous congestion/hypertension (clinically aggressive)
  - Second most common = carotid cavernous fistula (CCF)
    - Type A: Direct ICA-cavernous sinus shunt (not true dAVS)
    - Type B: Dural ICA branches-cavernous shunt
    - Type C: Dural ECA-cavernous shunt
    - Type D: ECA/ICA dural branches shunt to cavernous sinus
- MRA
  - TOF MRA may be negative with small or slow flow shunts or yield incomplete depiction of high flow lesions
  - Time resolved contrast augmented MRA useful for gross depiction of angioarchitecture and dynamics
  - PET/SPECT/perfusion MRI: May show increased rCBV, decreased rCBF (venous ischemia)

Imaging Recommendations
- Screening MR, contrast augmented MRA
- DSA to delineate vascular supply, venous drainage

Differential Diagnosis

Mixed Pial-Dural AVM
- True pial supply to dAVS is rare
- Usually occurs with large posterior fossa dAVS

Vascular Neoplasm
- Acutely thrombosed dAVS may enhance, have edema/mass effect

Pathology

General
- General Path Comments

- o No true nidus
- Etiology-Pathogenesis-Pathophysiology
  - o Most dAVSs are acquired
    - May be idiopathic
    - Can occur in response to trauma, venous occlusion, or venous hypertension
  - o Pathological activation of neoangiogenesis
    - Proliferating capillaries within granulation tissue in dural sinus obliterated by organized thrombi
    - Budding/proliferation of microvascular network in inner dura connects to plexus of thin-walled venous channels
    - High bFGF, VEGF expression in dAVSs
- Epidemiology
  - o 10-15% of all cerebrovascular malformations with AV shunting
  - o Location: Can occur anywhere but usually near skull base

Gross Pathologic or Surgical Features
- Multiple enlarged dural feeders converge on dural sinus
- Collection of "crack-like" vessels in wall of thrombosed sinus

Clinical Issues
Presentation
- Varies with age, location, severity of AV shunting
- Common
  - o Bruit, pulsatile tinnitus
  - o Exophthalmos
  - o Cranial neuropathy
- Uncommon
  - o Progressive dementia
  - o Parkinsonism
- Rare
  - o Life-threatening congestive heart failure
  - o Usually neonates, infants

Natural History
- Variable; can be aggressive with devastating hemorrhage
- Spontaneous closure rare

Treatment & Prognosis
- Endovascular
- Surgical resection
- Stereotaxic radiosurgery

Selected References
1. Kawaguchi T et al: Classification of venous ischaemia with MRI. J Clin Neurosci 8 (suppl 1): 82-8, 2001
2. Friedman JA et al: Results of combined stereotactic radiosurgery and transarterial embolization for dural arteriovenous fistulas of the transverse and sigmoid sinuses. J Neurosurg 94: 886-91, 2001
3. Uranishi R et al: Expression of angiogenic growth factors in dural arteriovenous fistula. J Neurosurg 91: 781-6, 1999

Carotid Cavernous Fistula

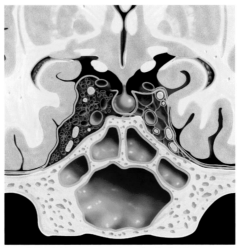

Note distension of the right cavernous sinus due to fistulous communication with internal carotid artery.

Key Facts
- Acronym: CCF
- Definition: Abnormal connection between internal carotid artery (ICA), cavernous sinus (CS)
- Classic imaging appearance
  - MR/CT: Exophthalmos with tortuosity and dilatation of superior ophthalmic veins
- Other key facts
  - Can be traumatic or spontaneous
  - Most common arteriovenous fistula (AVF) of the CNS
  - Rupture of ICA (direct) or its dural branches (indirect) results in sudden shunting of arterial blood into the CS
  - Dramatic orbital manifestations due to altered hemodynamics

Imaging Findings
General Features
- Dilated superior ophthalmic vein with enlarged cavernous sinus

CT/MR Findings
- Dilatation of superior ophthalmic vein (SOV)
- Exophthalmos with enlargement of extraocular muscles
- Enlarged cavernous sinus
  - Usually unilateral, occasionally bilateral (often asymmetric)
  - Imaging findings may not be present on studies early after traumatic episode

MRA/CTA Findings
- TOF MRA and CTA appearance can establish diagnosis
- Time-resolved contrast-augmented MRA depicts arterial shunting into sinus, early appearance of SOV

Angiography Findings
- Definitive for both diagnosis, therapy

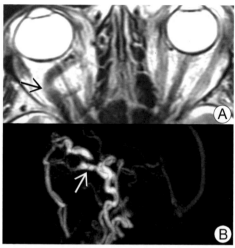

(A) Traumatic CCF: MR reveals bilateral proptosis with asymmetric dilatation of the SOV (arrow). (B) CCF: Time resolved contrast augmented MRA reveals rapid arterial phase shunting to the CS with filling of a dilated SOV (arrow).

- High flow direct CCFs may require injection into ipsilateral vertebral artery with manual compression of common carotid to demonstrate shunt site

Ultrasound
- Color Doppler shows flow reversal (intra- to extracranial) in enlarged SOV

Imaging Recommendations
- Screening U/S
- MR/MRA or CT/CTA to establish diagnosis or if presentation atypical but suspect
- Conventional DSA for definitive diagnosis and endovascular therapy
- Absence of dilated SOV or other imaging features does not exclude the diagnosis and should not preclude angiography

Differential Diagnosis: CCF

Thyroid Ophthalmopathy
- Most common cause of proptosis in adults
- 70% show clinical and biochemical evidence of hyperthyroidism
- Orbit findings bilateral in 80%
- Asymmetric involvement of extraocular muscles with inferior and medial rectus most common

Orbital Pseudotumor
- Idiopathic inflammatory condition of orbit
- Pain and inflammation usually evident
- Most common intraorbital mass in adults
- Steroid responsive

Cavernous Sinus Thrombosis/Thrombophlebitis
- Enlarged cavernous sinus and SOV on routine MRI
- Absence of flow void on routine MR, flow sensitive sequences confirm thrombosis
- May occur in association with CCF
- Fever and meningitis signal septic thrombophlebitis

- May see thrombus in CS on CT or MR

Pathology

General

- Etiology-Pathogenesis
  - Rupture of cavernous carotid or its dural branches into cavernous sinus results in altered regional hemodynamics
  - Valveless orbital veins transmit increased venous pressure resulting in orbital venous hypertension, venous distention, chemosis
  - Occurs spontaneously or after closed head injury and basilar skull fracture (may have delayed presentation)
  - Spontaneous CCF (usually indirect) occurs most often in middle-aged females

Clinical Issues

Presentation

- Classic = pulsatile exophthalmos, chemosis with persistent bruit (strongly suggests diagnosis)
- Typically occurs weeks to months after a traumatic episode
- May present with partial or complete III–VI cranial nerve palsies

Natural History

- Eyes at risk due to the potential of ocular necrosis

Treatment

- Endovascular therapy with embolization

Prognosis

- Treatment aimed at symptom relief with 90% success

Selected References
1. Accreditation Council on Graduate Medical Education: Arteriovenous fistulae of the CNS. AJNR 22(Suppl): S22-S25, 2001
2. Phatouros CC et al: Carotid artery cavernous fistulas. Neurosurg Clin N Am 11(1): 67-84, 2000
3. Coskun O et al: Carotid-cavernous fistulas: Diagnosis with spiral CT angiography. AJNR 22(4): 712-6, 2000

Hemangioblastoma

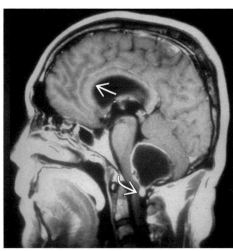

Contrast-enhanced T1WI demonstrates cystic cerebellar mass with enhancing nodule (curved arrow) in a 42-year-old man presenting with headaches due to obstructive hydrocephalus (upward bowing of corpus callosum - arrow).

Key Facts
- Most common posterior fossa intra-axial mass in middle-aged/older adult = metastasis, **not** hemangioblastoma (HGB)
- 75% of HGBs are sporadic; 25% occur with Von Hippel-Lindau (VHL) disease

Imaging Findings
General Features
- Von Hippel-Lindau disease associated tumor
- 60% cyst + "mural" nodule; 40% solid
- Best diagnostic sign = cystic mass with enhancing mural nodule abutting pia

CT Findings
- NECT: Low density cyst + isodense nodule
- CECT
  - Common: Nodule enhances strongly, uniformly; cyst doesn't
  - Less common: Solid tumor
  - Rare: Ring-enhancing mass

MR Findings
- Sensitivity of MR >> CT for small HGBs
- Cyst hypo-, nodule isointense with brain on T1WI
- Hyperintense on T2WI
- Prominent "flow voids" in some cases
- Nodule enhances strongly, intensely

Other Modality Findings
- DSA: Large avascular mass (cyst) + highly vascular nodule (prolonged blush, sometimes A-V shunting)
- Thallium-201 SPECT shows fast washout

Imaging Recommendations
- Begin MRI screening of patients from VHL families after age 11y
- Scan spinal cord with contrast for coexisting HGB

Hemangioblastoma

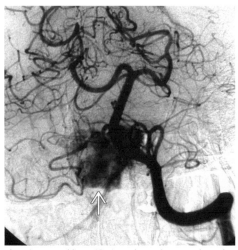

Left vertebral angiogram, oblique AP view, shows dense, prolonged vascular stain characteristic of hemangioblastoma (arrow).

Differential Diagnosis

Metastasis
- Most common parenchymal posterior fossa mass in middle-aged, older adults
- Usually not as vascular as HGB

Glioma
- Very rare posterior fossa mass in older adults

Other
- Clear cell ependymoma

Pathology

General
- General Path Comments
  - VHL phenotypes
    - Type 1 = without pheochromocytoma
    - Type 2A = with pheochromocytoma, renal cell carcinoma (RCC)
    - Type 2B = with pheochromocytoma, without RCC
- Genetics
  - Familial HGB (VHL disease)
    - Autosomal dominant
    - Chromosome 3p mutation
    - Suppressor gene product (VHL protein) causes neoplastic transformation
    - VEGF highly expressed in stromal cells
    - Other VHL gene mutations common
  - Sporadic HGB
    - Upregulation of erythropoietin common in both sporadic, VHL-related HGB
- Etiology-Pathogenesis-Pathophysiology
  - Unknown origin
- Epidemiology

Hemangioblastoma

- o 2% of primary CNS tumors
  - 7-10% of posterior fossa tumors
  - Rare: Supratentorial (usually along optic pathways)
- o 3-13% of spinal cord tumors
- o 75% of HGB are sporadic; 25% associated with VHL

Gross Pathologic or Surgical Features
- Well-circumscribed, highly vascular nodule +/- cyst

Microscopic Features
- Cyst wall usually compressed brain, not neoplasm
- Nodule = large, vacuolated stromal cells + rich capillary network

Staging or Grading Criteria
- WHO grade I

Clinical Issues

Presentation
- Sporadic HGB
  - o 40-60 y
  - o Headache (85%), dysequilibrium, dizziness
- Familial
  - o VHL-associated HGBs occur at younger age but are rare < 15y
  - o Retinal HGB
    - Ocular hemorrhage often first manifestation of VHL
    - Mean onset 25y
  - o Other: Symptoms due to RCC, polycythemia, endolymphatic sac tumor

Natural History
- Benign tumor with slow growth pattern
- Two-thirds with one VHL-associated HGB develop additional lesions
  - o Average = one new lesion every 2 years
  - o Require period screening, lifelong follow-up

Treatment & Prognosis
- Surgical resection +/- pre-operative embolization
  - o 85% 10 year survival rate
  - o 15-20% recurrence rate
  - o Median life expectancy in VHL = 49 years

Selected References
1. Conway JE et al: Hemangioblastomas of the CNS in von Hippel-Lindau syndrome and sporadic disease. Neurosurg 48: 55-63, 2001
2. Kondo T et al: Diagnostic value of ^{201}Tl-single-photon emission computerized tomography studies in cases of posterior fossa hemangioblastomas. J Neurosurg 95: 292-7, 2001
3. Bohling T et al: von Hippel-Lindau disease and capillary hemangioblastoma. In Kleihues P, Cavenee WK (eds): Tumours of the Nervous System, 223-6, IARC Press, 2000

Migraine

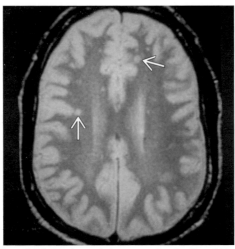

Multiple white matter lesions (arrows) shown on proton density weighted image in a patient with migraine headaches.

Key Facts
- Synonyms: "Vascular headache," cluster headache
- Definition: Unilateral severe headache preceded by scintillating scotomata
- Classic imaging appearance: Punctate white matter lesions in centrum semiovale on T2WI
- MR perfusion imaging can demonstrate hypoperfusion, typically in occipital lobes during acute attack
- MR diffusion imaging may be positive when hemiplegic or hemisensory symptoms are (or have recently been) present
- Cortical infarcts may be seen rarely

Imaging Findings
General Features
- Best imaging clue: Deep white matter lesions on T2WI in 5-12%
CT Findings
- NECT: Generally none
- CECT: Generally none
MR Findings
- T1WI: Generally none; rarely cortical infarcts
- T2WI: **Punctate hyperintensity** in centrum semiovale
- Perfusion imaging: May demonstrate decreased perfusion in occipital lobes during acute attack
- Diffusion and perfusion imaging: May be positive if focal neurologic deficits present
Other Modality Findings
- DSA: Increased incidence of cervical dissection
Imaging Recommendations
- MRI (FLAIR) may show punctate hyperintensities in deep white matter

Migraine

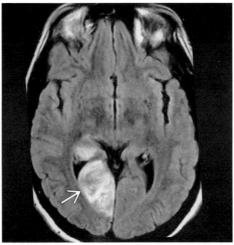

Complicated migraine in a 32-year-old woman with long history of migraines. This FLAIR image was taken 6 days after she presented with left homonymous hemianopsia and demonstrates presumed infarction (arrow) in the right PCA territory. (Courtesy M. Brant-Zawadzki MD)

Differential Diagnosis

Multiple Sclerosis
- Clinically not associated with headaches but rather remitting neurologic sx
- 2 mm sagittal FLAIR images demonstrate subcallosal striations oriented perpendicular to ependyma

Deep White Matter Ischemia
- Typically older patients or those with hypertension, diabetes, or hyperlipidemia

Vasculitis
- Cortical and deep white matter infarcts and occasional hemorrhage

Pathology

General
- Classically vasoconstriction of calcarine artery (leading to scintillating scotomata) followed by vasodilatation (leading to headache)
- Genetics
  - Familial migraine may be related to the CACNA1A gene
- Epidemiology
  - Affects 15-30% of population
  - More common in women
  - Often familial

Gross Pathologic or Surgical Features
- Rarely can produce cortical infarcts

Microscopic Features
- Gliosis in deep white matter from presumed small vessel infarction

Clinical Issues

Presentation
- "Common" migraine: 80% of cases

Migraine

- o Unilateral, throbbing, severe headache
- "Classic" migraine: 10% of cases
  - o **Headache** preceded by **aura** of sensory, motor, or visual symptoms ("scintillating scotomata") lasting 30 minutes or less
- "Complicated" migraine
  - o Neurologic deficits last longer than 30 minutes (or permanent)
- "Ophthalmic" migraine: Scintillating scotomata without headache or neurologic deficits (common)

Treatment
- Ergot derivatives, e.g., dihydroergotamine mesylate
- Serotonin receptor agonists, e.g., sumatriptan
- Analgesics

Prognosis
- Variable, painful but not fatal

Selected References
1. Osborn RE et al: MR imaging of the brain in patients with migraine headaches. AJNR 12: 521-4, 1991
2. Soges LJ et al: Migraine: evaluation of MR. AJNR 9: 425-9, 1988
3. Tatemichi TK et al: Migraine and stroke. In Barnett HJM, et al, eds: Stroke, pathophysiology, diagnosis and management, Vol 2, New York, Churchill Livingstone, 1986

Superficial Siderosis

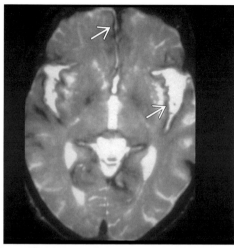

74-year-old man with multiple previous subarachnoid hemorrhages now with increasing sensorineural hearing loss. Leptomeninges appear outlined in black (arrows) on this T2W image due to hemosiderin deposition.

Key Facts
- Synonym: Siderosis
- Definition: Hemosiderin staining of leptomeninges following repeated SAH
- Classic imaging appearance: Surface of brain appears to be outlined in black on T2WI
- Generally causes deafness and ataxia

Imaging Findings
General Features
- Best imaging clue: Black outline of brain on T2WI
CT Findings
- Cerebral atrophy
- Slightly hyperdense rim over brain surface
MR Findings
- T2WI: Dark border on local surface of brain
- T2*WI (GRE): Most sensitive; FSE least sensitive
Imaging Recommendations
- T2W MRI initially identifies diagnosis
- T2*: Can be used to verify diagnose

Differential Diagnosis
Normal Leptomeningeal Melanin Deposition in African Americans
- No symptoms
Fast Spin Echo Artifact
- Worse on FSE than T2*W GRE

Pathology
General
- Hemosiderin staining of meninges
  - Hemosiderin is cytotoxic to underlying tissues

Superficial Siderosis

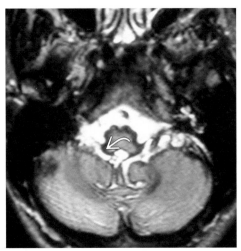

47-year-old man with hearing loss and ataxia following previous subarachnoid hemorrhages. Brainstem (curved arrow) and cerebellum appear outlined in black due to hemosiderin deposition in leptomeninges.

- Xanthochromic CSF
- Etiology-Pathogenesis
  - Repeated SAH
  - Hemosiderin is toxic to neurons
  - 8th CN is extensively lined with CNS myelin which is supported by hemosiderin-sensitive microglia
    - Increased exposure in pontine cistern
  - MR findings do not correlate with severity of disease

Gross Pathologic or Surgical Features
- Dark brown discoloration of leptomeninges, ependyma, and subpial tissue
- Causes
  - CSF cavity lesion with fragile neovascularity most common
  - Bleeding neoplasms (35%: Ependymoma, oligodendroglioma, astrocytoma)
  - Vascular abnormalities (18%)
    - Arteriovenous malformation (AVM), aneurysm
    - Multiple cavernous malformation near brain surface
  - Traumatic cervical nerve root avulsion
  - Idiopathic in 46%

Microscopic Features
- Hemosiderin staining of meninges and subpial tissues to 3 mm depth
- Thickened leptomeninges
- Cerebellar folia: Loss of Purkinje cells and Bergmann gliosis

Clinical Issues
Presentation
- Most common symptom: Bilateral sensorineural hearing loss (95% of cases),
- Other symptoms
  - Ataxia (88%)

- o Bilateral hemiparesis (76%), hyperreflexia
- o Bladder disturbance
- o Anosmia, dementia
- o Headache (30%)

Natural History
- Profound bilateral sensorineural hearing loss within 15 years of onset
- M:F ratio = 3:1

Treatment
- Surgically remove source of bleeding (surgical cavity, tumor, AVM)

Prognosis
- Deafness almost certain

Selected References
1. Spetzler RF et al: Modified classification of spinal cord vascular lesions. J Neurosurg (Spine 2) 96: 145-56, 2002
2. Bemporad JA et al: Magnetic resonance imaging of spinal cord vascular malformations with an emphasis on the cervical spine. In Neuropathic basis for imaging. Neuroimaging Clinics of North America 11: 111-29, 2001
3. Bao YH et al: Classification and therapeutic modalities of spinal vascular malformations in 80 patients. Neurosurgery 40: 75-81, 1997

Hypertensive Hemorrhage

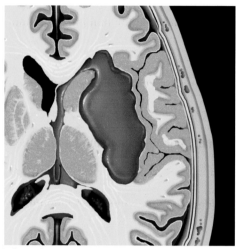

Axial graphic depicts hypertensive basal ganglionic hemorrhage with dissection into the lateral ventricle. Hematoma epicenter is lateral putamen/external capsule.

Key Facts
- Hypertension (HTN) most common cause of spontaneous intracranial hemorrhage (ICH) between 45-70 years
- Ganglionic bleed is most common pattern
- Chronic HTN may cause multifocal "black dots" on T2WI, T2* scans

Imaging Findings
<u>General Features</u>
- Two distinct patterns seen with hypertensive hemorrhage
  - Acute focal hematoma
  - Multiple subacute/chronic "microbleeds"
  - Best diagnostic sign = **putamen hematoma** in patient with HTN

<u>CT Findings</u>
- Elliptical high density mass
  - Most common = between putamen, insular cortex
  - Other sites = thalamus, pons
- Mixed density if coagulopathy, active bleeding
- Other: Hydrocephalus, IVH, herniation

<u>MR Findings</u>
- In primary intracranial hemorrhage group
- Contrast extravasation = active hemorrhage, growing hematoma
- Multifocal hypointense lesions on T2*
  - Common with longstanding HTN
  - Also seen with amyloid angiopathy

<u>Other Modality Findings</u>
- DSA/CTA
  - Almost always normal if HTN + deep ganglionic hemorrhage
  - May show avascular mass effect

<u>Imaging Recommendations</u>
- NECT scan

Hypertensive Hemorrhage

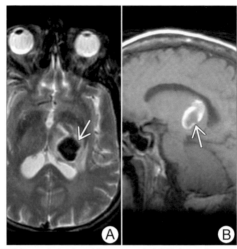

(A) Axial T2WI demonstrates hypointense mass in left thalamus (arrow). (B) Sagittal T1WI is hyperintense peripherally & isointense centrally (arrow), indicating acute-early subacute hematoma with intracellular deoxyhemoglobin centrally & intracellular methemoglobin peripherally.

- If older patient with HTN, typical hematoma, stop
- If no clear cause of hemorrhage or atypical appearance, consider MR (include contrast-enhanced, T2* sequences) + MRA
- If MR shows co-existing multifocal "black dots," stop
- If MR shows atypical hematoma, CTA
- If CTA inconclusive, consider DSA

Differential Diagnosis
Basal Ganglionic Hemorrhage
- Vascular malformation (younger patients)
- Hemorrhagic neoplasm (often mixed signal, enhancing)
- Other: Coagulopathy, drug abuse

Lobar Hemorrhage
- Amyloid angiopathy (elderly, demented, normotensive; rarely involves deep subcortical nuclei)
- Thrombosed AVM or dural arteriovenous shunt (dAVS) (younger patients with stagnating vessels, early draining veins on angiography)
- Cortical vein thrombosis (co-existing dural sinus thrombosis often - but not always - present)

Multifocal "Black Dots"
- Hemorrhagic diffuse axonal injury (DAI)
- Multiple cavernous/capillary malformations
- Amyloid angiopathy

Pathology
General
- General Path Comments (location)
  - Striatocapsular (putamen/external capsule) 60-65%
  - Thalamus 15-25%
  - Pons, cerebellum 10%

Hypertensive Hemorrhage

- o Lobar 5-15%
- o Multifocal "microbleeds" 1-5%
- Etiology-Pathogenesis
  - o "Bleeding globe" (penetrating artery aneurysm)
  - o Chronic HTN with atherosclerosis, fibrinoid necrosis, abrupt wall rupture +/- pseudoaneurysm formation
  - o NB: 10-15% of hypertensive patients with spontaneous ICH have underlying aneurysm or AVM
- Epidemiology
  - o 50% of primary ICHs caused by hypertensive hemorrhage

Gross Pathologic or Surgical Features
- Large ganglionic hematoma +/- intraventricular hemorrhage (IVH)
- Subfalcine herniation, hydrocephalus common
- Co-existing small, chronic hemorrhages, ischemic lesions common

Microscopic Features
- Fibrous balls (fibrosed miliary aneurysm)
- Severe arteriosclerosis with hyalinization, pseudoaneurysm
  - o Lacks media
  - o Lacks internal elastic lamina

Clinical Issues
Presentation
- Large ICHs present with sensorimotor deficits, impaired consciousness
- Seasonal, diurnal blood pressure variations cause higher incidence of ICH in colder months

Natural History
- Bleeding can persist for up to 6h following ictus
- Neurologic deterioration common within 48h
  - o Increasing hematoma
  - o Edema
  - o Development of hydrocephalus
  - o Herniation syndromes
- Recurrent hypertensive hemorrhage (hICH) in 5-10% of cases, usually different location

Treatment & Prognosis
- Prognosis related to location, size of ICH
- 80% mortality in massive ICH with IVH
- One-third of survivors are severely disabled
- Stereotaxic evacuation may improve outcome

Selected References
1. Chung CS et al: Striatocapsular haemorrhage. Brain 123: 1850-62, 2000
2. Broderick JP et al: Guidelines for the management of spontaneous intracerebral hemorrhage. Stroke 30: 905-15, 1999
3. Tanaka A et al: Small chronic hemorrhages and ischemic lesions in association with spontaneous intracerebral hematomas. Stroke 30: 1637-42, 1999

EC-IC Bypass

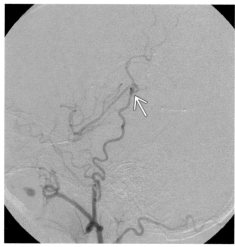

Left common carotid angiogram, arterial phase, lateral view, in a patient with an occluded cervical ICA and superficial temporal to MCA bypass (arrow). (Courtesy Anne G Osborn MD)

Key Facts
- Definition: Surgical anastomosis between external carotid artery (ECA) and internal carotid artery (ICA)
- Classic imaging appearance
  - Craniotomy with superficial temporal artery connected to ipsilateral medial cerebral artery (MCA)
- ICA occlusion
  - May lead to multilobar infarction and serious neurological injury
  - May produce only TIA, minor cerebrovascular accident (CVA) or be incidental finding
  - Clinical consequences dependent on patency of collateral channels including
    - Circle of Willis
    - External carotid artery
    - Pial vasculature
- Treatment options for ICA occlusion
  - Endarterectomy not effective with ICA occlusion
  - Medical treatment with anticoagulants and antiplatelet agents
  - Bypass option may be taken in those with altered perfusion
    - Identification of subgroup with PET, SPECT or perfusion MR/CT

Imaging Findings: ICA Occlusion/ EC-IC Bypass
<u>General Features</u>
- Best imaging clue: Absent ICA flow void on MRI
<u>CT Findings</u>
- CECT
  - Absent enhancement of ICA
  - Vascular tangle bridging ECA and MCA in post craniotomy patient
  - CTA delineates bypass anatomy

EC-IC Bypass

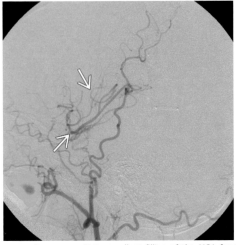

Same case as previous page. Note excellent filling of the MCA from the EC-IC anastomosis (arrow). (Courtesy Anne G Osborn MD)

MRI Findings
- MRI
  - Absent flow void, atypical intravascular hyperintensity seen with slow flow and occlusion of ICA
  - 2D flow sensitive sequences most specific for occlusion
- MRA
  - 2D TOF superior to 3D techniques in differentiating slow flow from occlusion
  - Black blood techniques may be helpful in confirming occlusion

Perfusion MRI/CT
- Reduced cerebral blood flow
- Prolonged MTT
- Compensatory elevation of cerebral blood volume, or reduction due to failed autoregulation
- Worsening with diamox challenge = poor prognostic sign

Other Modality Findings
- PET/SPECT may reveal ischemia

Imaging Recommendations
- Bypass patency can be established/monitored with noninvasive CTA/MRA
- Assessment for ischemia with perfusion CT/MR

Pathology
General
- ICA occlusion generally due to ASVD
- Bypass also done in patients with skull base pathology (tumors, aneurysms) unable to tolerate required carotid sacrifice

Clinical Issues
Presentation
- ICA occlusion symptomatology ranges from incidental finding to acute CVA

- Ongoing ischemia with best medical therapy forces consideration of bypass

Prognosis
- Poor in ischemic group with ICA occlusion without bypass procedure
- Survival rate very high beyond perioperative period

Selected References
1. Guthikonda M et al: Future of extracranial-intracranial bypass. Neurol Res 24 Suppl1: 80-3, 2002
2. Grubb RI et al: Importance of hemodynamic factors in the prognosis of symptomatic carotid occlusion. JAMA 280: 1055-60, 1998
3. The EC/IC Bypass Study group: Failure of extracranial-intracranial arterial bypass to reduce the risk of ischemic stroke: Results of an international randomized trial. N Engl J Med 313: 1191-200, 1985

Primary Intracranial Hemorrhage

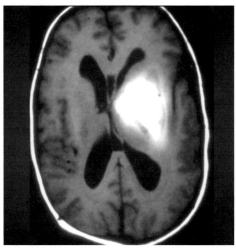

T1WI demonstrates subacute hematoma in left basal ganglia with mass effect.

Key Facts
- Nontraumatic primary intracranial hemorrhage (pICH) causes 15-20% of acute "strokes"
- Hypertension (HTN), cerebral amyloid angiopathy (CAA), coagulopathy most common causes of pICH in elderly
- Patients < 45y often have underlying vascular lesion such as aneurysm, cerebral vascular malformation (CVM), venous occlusion

Imaging Findings
General Features
- Best diagnostic signs
  - Deep (ganglionic) hematoma in HTN
  - Lobar/subcortical hematoma in CAA, CVM,
  - If unilateral, possible venous occlusion ("venous infarct")
  - If bilateral, posterior, parasagittal, possible SSS thrombosis
CT Findings
- Round/elliptical parenchymal mass
  - Acute ICH usually hyperdense (from 1 hour to about 3-5 days)
  - May be mixed iso-/hyperdense if rapid bleeding, coagulopathy
  - Peripheral low density (vasogenic edema)
- Ganglionic ICH may extend into lateral ventricle
MR Findings
- Signal from pICH varies with numerous factors including
  - MR technique, e.g., sensitivity to magnetic susceptibility effects (T2* shortening): GRE > CSE > FSE
  - Type of contrast: T2*WI > T2WI > T1WI
  - Location: Parenchymal, intraventricular, subdural, epidural, SAH
  - Form of hemoglobin: OxyHgb, deoxyHgb, metHgb, hemachromes/hemosiderin
  - RBC lysis, paramagnetism of heme Fe, surrounding edema
- 5 stages of hemorrhage (need both T1WI and T2WI)

Primary Intracranial Hemorrhage

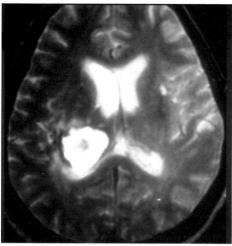

T2WI demonstrates chronic hematoma (central extracellular methemoglobin surrounded by hemosiderin) in right thalamus extending into right lateral ventricle. Both patients (this image and the image on the previous page) were hypertensive.

- **Hyperacute** (< 24 hours): Core-intracellular oxyHgb (hypointense on T1WI, hyperintense on T2WI); border-intracellular deoxyHgb (dark on T2WI)
  - "DeoxyHgb border sign": Appears almost immediately on T2WI
  - More sensitive for parenchymal hemorrhage and sooner than CT
- **Acute** (1-3 days), intracellular deoxyHgb, dark on T2WI (darkest on T2* w-GRE, least dark on T2W-FSE)
- **Early subacute** (3-7 days), intracellular metHgb, bright on T1WI, dark on T2WI
- **Late subacute** (7-14 days), extracellular metHgb, bright on both T1WI and T2WI
- **Chronic** (14 + days; parenchymal hematomas only)
  - Core: Bright extracellular metHgb becoming hemachromes (proteinaceous heme derivatives) over months
  - Rim: Hemosiderin and ferritin (dark on T2WI)

Other Modality Findings
- DSA: May show AVM, vasculitis, aneurysm, or tumor
- PET: May be useful for neoplastic vs. nonneoplastic etiology

Imaging Recommendations
- NECT: If hematoma/history typical for HTN or trauma and normal: Stop
- If atypical hematoma or unclear history, do T1W and T2*W MRI followed by T1W with gadolinium
- DSA if suspicious for vasculitis

Differential Diagnosis
HTN vs. CAA (see "Cerebral Amyloid Angiopathy")
- Both occur in older patients
- Both may have evidence of previous hemorrhages
- HTN usually ganglionic; amyloid usually subcortical and lobar

Primary Intracranial Hemorrhage

- Amyloid usually > 70y, normotensive, demented

Hypertensive Bleed vs. Neoplasm, Vascular Malformation
- HTN unusual in young patients unless drug abuse (e.g., cocaine)
- Neoplasm often has disordered evolution of hemorrhage, foci of contrast enhancement

Cortical Vein Thrombosis
- Adjacent dural sinus often (but not always) thrombosed

Pathology
General
- Etiology-Pathogenesis-Pathophysiology
  - Older patients
    - Basal ganglionic = HTN
    - Lobar = amyloid angiopathy
    - Neoplasm (2-14% of "spontaneous" ICH)
    - Coagulopathy
    - Venous occlusion, vascular malformation, aneurysm
  - Younger patients
    - Lobar = CVM
    - Other: Drug use, vasculitis, venous thrombosis

Gross Pathologic or Surgical Features
- Acute ganglionic/lobar hematoma

Microscopic Features
- Co-existing microangiopathy common in amyloid, HTN

Clinical Criteria
- Clinical ICH score correlates with
  - Admission GCS
  - Age > 80y, ICH volume
  - Infratentorial
  - Presence of intraventricular hemorrhage (IVH)
  - 30-day mortality

Clinical Issues
Presentation
- > 50% of patients with pICH do not have HTN
- 90% of patients with recurrent pICH are hypertensive

Natural History
- Hematoma enlargement common in first 24-48h
  - Risk factors = EtOH, low fibrinogen, coagulopathy, irregularly shaped hematoma, disturbed consciousness
- 30% of patients rebleed within 1 year

Treatment & Prognosis
- Mortality 30-55% in first month
- Surgical evacuation controversial
- Recovery poor; most survivors have significant deficits

Selected References
1. Linfante I et al: MRI features of intracerebral hemorrhage within 2 hours from symptom onset. Stroke 30: 2263-7, 1999
2. Atlas SW et al: MR Detection of hyperacute parenchymal hemorrhage of the brain. AJNR 19: 1471-7, 1998
3. Bradley WG: MR appearance of hemorrhage in the brain. Radiology 189: 15-26, 1993

Post-Op Aneurysm

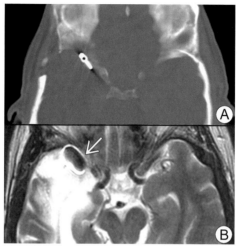

NECT scan after (A) clipping of the right MCA aneurysm 12 years prior to imaging shows metallic clip. (B) T2WI shows encephalomalacia, clip artifact (arrow). (Courtesy Anne G Osborn MD)

Key Facts
- Synonym: Clipped aneurysm
- Definition: Metallic clip placed at neck of aneurysm intraoperatively
  - Potential complications: Subarachnoid hemorrhage (SAH), regrowth or new aneurysms, hydrocephalus, stroke
  - Potential dangers of MR imaging post-op aneurysms
- Classic imaging appearance: Metallic clip adjacent to blood vessel on angiography (A/G)
- Other key facts: **Potential danger**
  - MRI: If clip is ferromagnetic, it will torque in the magnetic field and can separate from the vessel, leading to SAH and likely death
    - Extremely important to screen patients with possible ferromagnetic aneurysm clips before MRI
    - History of type of aneurysm used in clipping may not be reliable
    - Important to verify with neurosurgeon directly type of clip used and to confirm with plain film if necessary
    - If clip is nonferromagnetic, MRI can be performed safely but there will be local image distortion
  - Short term follow up is important because of potential post-op complications
    - SAH, vasospasm, infarction, hydrocephalus, hemorrhage
  - Long term follow up is important because of regrowth of aneurysm and because incidence of de novo aneurysm formation higher after first one

Imaging Findings
General Features
- Best imaging clue for routine follow up: Metallic clip next to vessel on A/G
- Best imaging for complications
  - SAH: Use MRI (CSF bright on FLAIR)

Post-Op Aneurysm

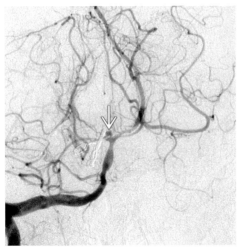

Right vertebral DSA, AP view, after clipping of basilar bifurcation aneurysm. Note vasospasm, neck remnant (arrow). (Courtesy Anne G Osborn MD)

- o Vasospasm: Use A/G to show luminal narrowing
- o Stroke: Use diffusion imaging (bright)
- o Communicating hydrocephalus: MRI

CT Findings
- NECT: Metallic artifact arising from clip; SAH will appear as bright CSF

MR Findings
- T1WI and T2WI: Metallic artifact arising from clip
  - o Ferromagnetic clip: Large artifact (50% of head size)
  - o Nonferromagnetic clip: Small artifact (2-3 cm)
  - o To minimize artifact: Use FSE and increase bandwidth
- MRA of limited value due to metallic artifact (use DSA)
- If SAH suspected: Use FLAIR
  - o 100% sensitive for acute SAH (more sensitive than CT)
  - o Less than 100% specificity, e.g., meningitis, CSF inflow
- If vasospasm suspected, could be missed on MRA (use DSA)
- If stroke suspected, use diffusion imaging

Trans-Cranial Doppler Findings
- Velocity > 120 cm/sec in the M1 segment of the MCA indicates vasospasm

Imaging Recommendations
- For routine follow up of post-op aneurysm or de novo formation: DSA
- For suspected SAH: FLAIR or CT
- For suspected vasospasm: TCD then A/G
- For suspected stroke: Diffusion imaging
- CTA/MRA may be useful to detect abnormalities occult to conventional angiography, particularly with conventional biplane techniques
- Knowledge of clip ferromagnetic properties essential before consideration for MR imaging; GDC coils are MR safe

Differential Diagnosis
Subarachnoid Hemorrhage
- Bright CSF on FLAIR; DDx

- o CSF inflow (flow-related enhancement)
- o Meningitis (protein leakage causing T1 shortening and lack of nulling by initial inversion pulse in FLAIR)

Vasospasm
- DDx: Vasculitis, intracranial arteriosclerosis

Pathology

General
- General Path Comments
  - o SAH reported after surgical clipping in 1-2% of patients
    - 70% develop vasospasm
    - 20-40% develop focal neurologic defects due to spasm
    - Amount of SAH on initial CT predictive for delayed ischemia and infarction
    - Vasospasm decreased if SAH removed surgically within 48-72h
  - o Regrowth of completely clipped aneurysms is 0.26% annually
  - o Regrowth of incompletely clipped aneurysms is approx 1% annually
  - o De novo aneurysm formation after clipping is 0.89% annually
- Anatomy
  - o Most clipped aneurysms are near the Circle of Willis

Surgical Features
- Aneurysm clip becomes functional wall of vessel
  - o Different from hemoclips which can be scanned safely since are on clipped side branches which subsequently clot – not functional wall

Clinical Issues

Presentation
- SAH: "Worst headache of my life"
- Stroke: Focal neurologic symptoms
- Regrowth or de novo aneuysm: New cranial nerve palsy or headache

Natural History
- 1-2% will develop SAH post clipping
  - o About one third of these will develop focal neurologic symptoms as a result
- 1% will have regrowth of the clipped aneurysm or develop new ones
- Patients should insist on use of nonferromagnetic clips and carry evidence of such if MRI ever required for any reason

Treatment
- SAH can be surgically removed to decrease chance of stroke
- New aneurysms can be clipped or coiled

Prognosis
- Ongoing risk of SAH and regrowth of clipped aneurysm or appearance of new aneurysms
- Greater chance of stroke due to SAH
- Risk of death from MRI if ferromagnetic clip used

Selected References
1. Hohlrieder M et al: Cerebral vasospasm and ischemic infarction in clipped and coiled intracranial aneurysm patients. Eur J of Neurology 9: 389-99, 2002
2. Tsutsumi K et al: Risk of aneurysm recurrence in patients with clipped cerebral aneurysms. Stroke 32: 1191-4, 2001
3. Kivisaari RP et al: MR imaging after aneurysmal subarachnoid hemorrhage and surgery: A long-term follow-up study. AJNR 22: 1143-8, 2001

PocketRadiologist™
Vascular
Top 100 Diagnoses

HEAD & NECK

Carotid Stenosis, Extracranial

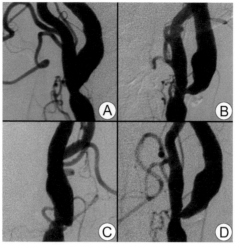

(A-D). 4 views of a common carotid DSA are shown. Maximum stenosis is profiled in (B).

Key Facts
- Stroke is the second most common worldwide cause of death
- Most cerebral infarcts occur in carotid vascular territory
- Carotid stenosis = 70% associated with significant stroke risk, benefit from endarterectomy

Imaging Findings
General Features
- Smooth or irregular narrowing, usually at internal carotid artery (ICA) origin
CT Findings
- +/- Ca++ in vessel wall
- Large plaques may show low-density foci
MR Findings
- MRA provides multidirectional imaging (vs. conventional DSA)
- "Flow gap" (recovery of signal) may render MRA non-diagnostic in high-grade stenosis
- Signal loss can occur in severely narrowed artery (> 95%) causing mis-diagnosis of occlusion
- Brain T2WI, FLAIR may show "rosary-like" lesions in centrum semiovale ipsilateral to stenosis (hemodynamic failure?)
Ultrasound (US) Findings
- High velocity flow in stenotic zone, proportionate to degree of narrowing
- Post-stenotic flow disturbance
- Pulsatility changes proximal and distal to severe stenosis
Other Modality Findings
- CTA
  - Demonstrates lumen narrowing
  - Wall Ca++ identified
  - Poor correlation with ulceration

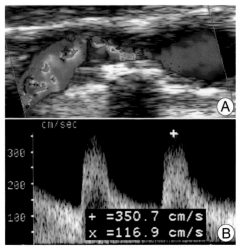

Ultrasound ICA stenosis. (A) Color Doppler image showing severe carotid narrowing and post-stenotic flow disturbance. (B) Doppler spectrum analysis documents high velocity flow consistent with 70% or greater ICA stenosis (peak systolic velocity 351 cm/sec, end diastolic velocity 117 cm/sec).

- o Patchy/homogeneous low density in wall often seen with large necrotic/lipid plaque
- DSA
  - o Current standard of reference (NB: Enhanced CTA, MRA adequate for evaluation of carotid stenosis)
  - o Role of DSA
    - ▪ Evaluate great vessel origins for stenosis/occlusion
    - ▪ Calculate % carotid stenosis
    - ▪ Depict presence of collateral flow (lower risk of stroke, TIA)
    - ▪ Identify "tandem" distal ICA stenosis (2% of cases)
    - ▪ Detect other lesions (e.g., aneurysm)
    - ▪ At least 4 projections (AP, lat, both obliques) recommended
- Calculating carotid stenosis
  - o Methods vary
  - o NASCET method: Normal post-stenosis lumen diameter minus least residual diameter ÷ **post-bulbar** ICA diameter × 100
- Irregular plaque surface = increased stroke risk on medical treatment at all degrees of stenosis
- "Pseudoocclusion"
  - o Very high-grade stenosis, slow antegrade "trickle" of blood flow
    - ▪ May be shown only on late phase of angiogram
    - ▪ Requires technical diligence for US identification
    - ▪ Potential misdiagnosis on non-contrast MRA
  - o Important because endarterectomy an option if ICA still patent
  - o High stroke risk

Imaging Recommendations
- Ultrasound as screening tool
- CTA/MRA for comprehensive cerebrovascular evaluation
- DSA if US/CTA/MRA are equivocal or show "occlusion"

Carotid Stenosis, Extracranial

Differential Diagnosis
Extrinsic Compressive Lesion (Rare)
- Carotid space neoplasm

Dissection
- Typically spares bulb, ICA origin (ASVD involves both)
- No Ca++

Pathology
General
- Significant ICA narrowing identified in 20-30% of carotid territory strokes (vs. 5-10% of general population)
- Etiology-Pathogenesis-Pathophysiology
  - Risk of stroke increases with stenosis severity
    - Artery-to-artery emboli primary cause of stroke
    - Larger plaques are complicated by hemorrhage, necrosis, disruption of fibrous cap and intima, causing embolization
    - Stenosis = indirect measure of plaque volume and potential for complicated plaque/embolization
  - Plaque composition and surface morphology also stroke risk factors
  - Hypoperfusion may cause "watershed" infarcts, possibly centrum semiovale lesions

Gross Pathologic Features
- See "Atherosclerosis"

Microscopic Features
- See "Atherosclerosis"

Clinical Issues
Presentation
- Transient hemispheric ischemia (TIA)
- Stroke (can be silent, permanent, or with recovery)
- Amaurosis fugax (transient, monocular embolic blindness)

Natural History
- Progressive

Treatment & Prognosis
- NASCET
  - Symptomatic stenosis = 70% benefits from endarterectomy
  - Symptomatic moderate stenosis (50-69%) also benefits from endarterectomy in selected cases
- ACAS
  - Asymptomatic patients benefit from endarterectomy with stenosis of 60%
  - But low benefit compared with 70%, stenosis
- Benefit of endarterectomy highly dependent on institutional surgical risk

Selected References
1. Randoux B et al: Carotid artery stenosis: Prospective comparison of CT, Gadolinium-enhanced MR, and conventional angiography. Radiology 220: 179-85, 2001
2. Rothwell PM et al: Interrelation between plaque surface morphology and degree of stenosis on carotid angiograms and the risk of ischemic stroke in patients with symptomatic carotid stenosis. Stroke 31: 615-21, 2000
3. Moneta GL et al: Correlation of North American symptomatic carotid endarterectomy trial (NASCET) angiographic definition of 70% to 99% internal carotid artery stenosis with duplex scanning. J Vasc Surg 17:152-9, 1993

Vertebrobasilar Insufficiency

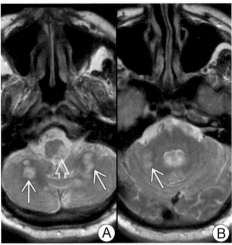

(A,B) Axial T2W images through posterior fossa demonstrating bilateral cerebellar infarcts (arrows) and left lateral medullary infarct (open arrow). Note absence of flow voids from either vertebral artery in basal cisterns indicating high-grade bilateral stenosis or occlusion.

Key Facts
- Synonyms: Vertebral artery stenosis, posterior circulation ischemia
- Definition: Posterior circulation ischemia of hemodynamic or embolic etiology
- Classic imaging appearance: Bilateral vertebral artery ostial stenosis
- Hemodynamic compromise (70% of cases)
  - Usually transient, postural or positional symptoms without stroke
- Embolic disease (30% of cases)
- Usually leads to debilitating, permanent infarcts

Imaging Findings
General Features
- Best imaging clue: Posterior circulation (occipital lobe, cerebellar or brainstem) stroke on MRI
CT Findings
- Focal atrophy of occipital lobe, cerebellum or brainstem
- Calcification of vertebral and/or basilar arteries
MR Findings
- T1WI and T2WI: Posterior circulation infarction
  - Acute: Mass effect in vascular territory
  - Subacute: No mass effect or atrophy; gyral enhancement with contrast or petechial hemorrhage on T2WI or T2*W-GRE
  - Chronic: Atrophy, sulcal enlargement
- Diffusion imaging: Bright if acute infarct, iso if subacute, dark if chronic
- Perfusion imaging: Decreased rCBV and rCBF and/or increased mean transit time (MTT) in posterior circulation vascular territory
- MRA
  - 3D TOF: Bilateral vertebral artery stenosis (> 70%) or basilar stenosis

Vertebrobasilar Insufficiency

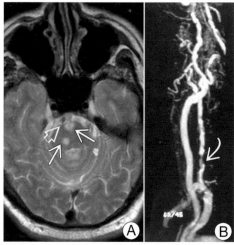

(A) Axial T2WI through pontine isthmus (same patient as previous page) shows R paramedian infarcts (arrows) & minimal flow void in basilar artery (open arrow) indicating slow flow. (B) Contrast-enhanced MRA of left vertebral artery shows diffuse irregularity due to multiple plaques & high-grade stenosis (curved arrow).

- If proximal subclavian stenosis: 2D TOF (from up to down & down to up) or posterior circulation MRA to show retrograde ipsilateral vertebral artery flow

Other Modality Findings
- DSA: Vertebrobasilar stenosis (> 70%) or proximal subclavian stenosis and retrograde flow in ipsilateral vertebral artery (subclavian steal)
- Transcranial Doppler ultrasound: Increased velocity in stenotic vertebrals

Imaging Recommendations
- MRA to evaluate subclavian, vertebral and basilar arteries

Differential Diagnosis
Cardiac Insufficiency
- No postural symptoms; no evidence subclavian, vertebral or basilar stenosis on MRA; CHF or arrhythmias
Overmedication with Antihypertensives
- Check drug levels
Anemia
- Check HCT
Brain Tumor
- Perform MRI
Benign Vertiginous State, e.g., Ménière's Labyrinthitis
Basilar Artery Migraine
Post-SAH Vasospasm
- Perform MRI (FLAIR) or angiogram (spasm)

Pathology
General
- General Path Comments: Vertebrobasilar insufficiency may be from hemodynamic or embolic causes

Vertebrobasilar Insufficiency

- Hemodynamic compromise (70% of cases)
  - If > 70% stenosis of both vertebral arteries and anterior circulation unable to compensate via circle of Willis
  - If > 70% subclavian stenosis proximal to origin of vertebral artery ("subclavian steal syndrome")
- Embolic disease (30% of cases)
  - From plaques or mural lesions of subclavian, vertebral or basilar artery
  - From atherosclerotic plaques, intimal defects, or (rarely) fibromuscular dysplasia, aneurysm or dissection
- Etiology-Pathogenesis
  - Atherosclerosis most common cause of both hemodynamic and embolic
  - Less common: Takayasu, fibromuscular dysplasia, trauma, osteophyte compression, dissection, aneurysm, other arteritides

Gross Pathologic or Surgical Features
- Stenosis of proximal subclavian artery, basilar artery, or both vertebral arteries and associated posterior circulation stroke

Clinical Issues

Presentation
- Hemodynamic compromise: Usually transient, postural or positional symptoms without stroke
- Embolic disease: Usually leads to debilitating, permanent infarcts
- Symptoms: Dizziness, vertigo, diplopia, dysarthria, perioral numbness, alternating paresthesias, tinnitus, dysphagia, drop attacks, ataxia, homonymous hemianopsia

Treatment
- Only indicated for symptomatic disease (vs. imaging diagnosis)
- Surgery: Depends on level of disease
  - Proximal subclavian stenosis (subclavian steal): Reconstruction
  - V1 (ostial lesions): Vertebral artery reconstruction or bypass to ipsilateral carotid or subclavian arteries
  - V2 (within cervical foramina): Check for compressing osteophytes
- Neurointerventional: Angioplasty and stent of subclavian, vertebral and basilar arteries (long term results still to be validated)
- Medical: Chronic anticoagulation

Prognosis
- If hemodynamic, little chance of stroke but trauma from fall likely
- If embolic, debilitating stroke likely without treatment
- With surgery, prognosis excellent

Selected References
1. Caplan L: Posterior circulation ischemia: Then, now, and tomorrow. Stroke 31: 2011-23, 2000
2. Berguer R et al: Surgical reconstruction of the extracranial vertebral artery: Management. J Vasc Surg 31: 9-18, 2000
3. Malek AM et al: Treatment of posterior circulation ischemia with extracranial percutaneous balloon angioplasty and stent placement. Stroke 30: 2073-85, 1999

Subclavian Steal

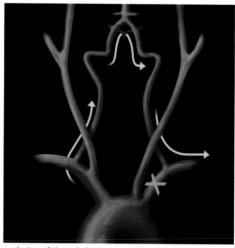

Stenosis or occlusion of the subclavian artery (at X) causes the upper extremity to "steal" blood from the ipsilateral vertebral artery.

Key Facts
- Synonym: Vertebral-to-subclavian steal
- Definition: Collateral blood flow to the arm via the vertebral arteries in response to subclavian artery stenosis or occlusion (see "Subclavian Stenosis and Occlusion")
- Classic imaging appearance
  - Reversed or biphasic vertebral artery (VA) flow ipsilateral to obstructed subclavian artery (SCA)
  - Antegrade VA flow contralateral to obstructed SCA
  - Increased volume/velocity of flow in contralateral VA
- Diminished arm pulses and blood pressure ipsilateral to SCA obstruction (arm-to-arm blood pressure difference of 20-30 mmHg)
- Generally a harmless, asymptomatic phenomenon, but can be symptomatic
- Predominately left side (85% of cases) but can occur on right

Imaging Findings
General Features
- Best imaging clue
  - VA flow reversal
  - SCA stenosis or occlusion
CTA/MRA/DSA Findings
- Flow is reversed or to-and fro in the affected VA and antegrade in contralateral VA
- High-grade SCA stenosis or occlusion ipsilateral to VA flow reversal
- **Note**: Flow reversal will be inapparent on 2D time-of-flight MR images but will be readily apparent on phase contrast images
Duplex Ultrasound Findings
- Reversed flow in the affected VA on color and spectral Doppler

Subclavian Steal

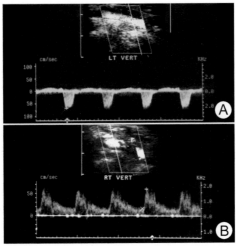

Doppler features of left subclavian steal. (A) In systole, blood flow is retrograde in the left VA (downward waveforms), with a small amount of antegrade flow in diastole. (B) Blood flow is antegrade in the right VA, with abnormally high velocity (peak systolic velocity = 60 cm/sec) caused by the collateral flow demand.

- Biphasic (to-and-fro) spectral Doppler flow in the affected VA at rest, with flow reversal following ipsilateral arm exercise (or tourniquet - induced hyperemia)
- Increased blood flow in the contralateral VA (not precisely defined, but peak systolic velocity > 60 cm/sec suggests abnormality)
- Damped Doppler waveforms (due to ischemia) in the affected SCA
- Possible Doppler evidence of SCA stenosis (focal high velocity, turbulence)

Imaging Recommendations
- Sonography to diagnose or confirm this condition
- MRA, CTA, or DSA for comprehensive pre-operative assessment

Differential Diagnosis
Right Common Carotid Steal
- Associated with high-grade innominate artery stenosis or occlusion (right side only)
- Analogous to subclavian steal, but blood is "stolen" from the right common carotid artery (RCCA), as well as the right VA
- To-and-fro or reversed RCCA and right VA flow

Pathology
General
- Atherosclerotic occlusive disease by far most common cause of SCA obstruction leading to subclavian steal
- Rarely, steal-inducing SCA obstruction may result from vasculitis, dissection, trauma, or a neoplastic mass
- Anatomy
  - Subclavian steal occurs because of unique VA anatomy, with the two VAs combining at the foramen magnum to form the basilar artery

o Blood flow is conveniently "stolen" from the ipsilateral VA, supplying the arm with collateral blood flow

Staging or Grading Criteria

- Persistent - the steal phenomenon is present at all times (implies SCA occlusion)
- Intermittent - the steal phenomenon occurs only when arm exercise increases blood flow demand (implies SCA stenosis)

Clinical Issues

Presentation

- Almost always a harmless, asymptomatic phenomenon
- Rarely causes vertebrobasilar stroke (even in presence of VA or carotid occlusive disease)
- If symptomatic
  o Arm claudication (pain with arm exercise)
  o Vertebrobasilar ischemic symptoms (classically dizziness) occurring with arm exercise

Prognosis

- Usually remains asymptomatic
- May become symptomatic with progression of atherosclerosis in the affected arm or the cerebral vasculature

Treatment

- Angioplasty/stent
- Common carotid-to-SCA bypass or innominate-to-SCA bypass

Selected References
1. Kliewer MA et al: Vertebral artery Doppler waveform changes indicating subclavian steal physiology. AJR 174: 815-9, 2000
2. Van Grimberge et al: The role of magnetic resonance in the diagnosis of subclavian steal syndrome. J Magn Reson Imaging 2: 339-42, 2000
3. Nicholls SC et al: Clinical significance of retrograde flow in the vertebral artery. Ann Vasc Surg 5: 331-6, 1991

Post-op Carotid Endarterectomy

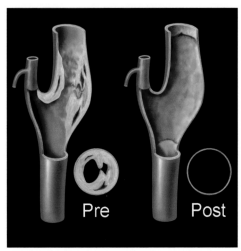

Pre: Diseased carotid bifurcation reveals significantly narrowed lumen due to extensive plaque with ulceration. Post: Post endarterectomy there is resection of intima-media complex and plaque resulting in a slightly wider than normal lumen.

Key Facts
- Definition: Surgical removal of atherosclerotic plaque from carotid bifurcation to alleviate flow-limiting stenosis
- Classic imaging appearance: Enlarged carotid bulb
- Imaging important to detect postoperative stroke and carotid restenosis

Imaging Findings
General Features
- Best imaging clue: Smoothly dilated carotid bulb and proximal ICA
CT Findings
- NECT: Metallic clips in the neck near the carotid bifurcation
- CTA: Dilated carotid bulb and proximal ICA with adjacent metallic clip artifact
MR Findings
- T1WI and T2WI of neck: Metallic artifact in the neck near carotid bifurcation
  - Metallic artifact minimized on high bandwidth FSE images
- T2WI and FLAIR of brain: Post-op infarction rarely
  - Diffusion positive acutely and may be positive with restenosis
- MRA: Metallic artifact near bifurcation may simulate restenosis
  - Important to evaluate source images to identify metallic artifact which is more subtle on MIP images
  - CEMRA better than nonenhanced
  - Metallic artifact minimized using higher bandwidth
Other Modality Findings
- Doppler U/S
  - Low ratio of ICA/CCA velocities
    - Usually means stenotic ICA (pre-op)
    - Due to low velocity in dilated CCA post-op
  - Can show residual plaque at endarterectomy site

Post-op Carotid Endarterectomy

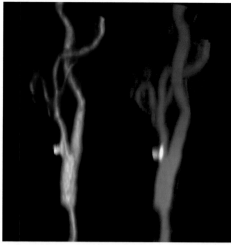

CTA performed to exclude acute carotid occlusion in a patient who became symptomatic in postoperative period demonstrates widened bifurcation and ICA. (Courtesy Lawrence N Tanenbaum MD)

- o TCD can demonstrate increased MCA flow post carotid endarterectomy (CEA)
- DSA: Normal – dilated smooth, tubular carotid bifurcation; abnormal: Restenosis, flap, web

Imaging Recommendations
- DSA for restenosis or other flow-limiting pathology

Differential Diagnosis
Fusiform Aneurysm of Carotid Bifurcation
- No history of CEA

Pathology
General
- General Path Comments
  - o Removal of plaque eliminates stenosis
- Epidemiology
  - o Women have a higher incidence of perioperative stroke than men
  - o Perioperative stroke and death rate post CEA at 30 days
    - ▪ 7.5% in ECST
    - ▪ 5.8% in NASCET
  - o Justified due to stroke risk reduction from CEA of
    - ▪ 9.6% in ECST
    - ▪ 17% in NASCET

Gross Surgical Features
- Two main CEA techniques
  - o Atherosclerotic plaque removed through arteriotomy
    - ▪ Closed with continuous vascular suture (smaller diameter, quicker surgery)
    - ▪ Closed with vein or synthetic patch (larger diameter, increases anesthesia time)("CEAP")

- o Carotid eversion endarterectomy (CEE)
  - Complete oblique transection of ICA at origin
  - Eversion of ICA upon itself
  - Complete removal of ICA plaque under direct visualization
  - End-to-side reimplantation of ICA more proximally on CCA
  - Shortening eliminates redundancy which can lead to thrombosis of ICA and perioperative stroke

Clinical Issues

Presentation
- Indication for CEA: **70% or greater** (flow-limiting) stenosis (by diameter, NASCET criteria)
- Risk factors for perioperative stroke
  - o Female sex
  - o Recent ipsilateral hemispheric stroke
  - o Contralateral carotid artery occlusion
  - o Left-sided CEA
  - o Plaque ulceration
  - o Age > 75 years
  - o Systolic BP > 180 mmHg
  - o Peripheral vascular disease
  - o Siphon or external carotid artery stenosis
  - o Cerebral ischemia (vs amaurosis fugax)
  - o Ipsilateral ischemic lesion on CT or MRI

Natural History
- Restenosis (50% narrowing) occurs 5-10%/year
  - o Not always symptomatic

Treatment for Restenosis
- Repeat CEA difficult due to fibrosis
- Angioplasty and stent preferred
- Aspirin

Prognosis
- Excellent if absent risk factors
- Good with risk factors: Mid and upper cervical ICA, infraforaminal vertebral arteries

Selected References
1. Ballotta E et al: Carotid eversion endarterectomy: Preoperative outcome and restenosis incidence. Ann Vasc Surg 16: 422-9, 2002
2. Trisal V et al: Carotid artery restenosis: An ongoing disease process. Am Surg 68: 275-9, 2002
3. Awad IA: Chapter 10: Cerebrovascular Occlusive Disease in Principles of Neurosurgery, Rengachary SS, Wilkins RH (Eds), Mosby, London, 10.2-10.20, 1994

Carotid Dissection

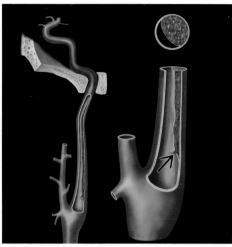

Graphic depicts subintimal dissection of the cervical internal carotid artery (ICA). Note proximal intimal tear (arrow), eccentric ICA narrowing. The bulb is spared and the dissection ends at the skull base.

Key Facts
- Definition: Delamination of wall of carotid artery from entry of blood (under arterial pressure) through a rent in intima
- Consider in young/middle-aged patient with headache, TIA, stroke (dissection causes 10-25% of ischemic strokes in young adults)
- CCA dissection: Usually an extension from arch dissection
- ICA dissection: Localized, most frequent site of head/neck dissection

Imaging Findings
General Features
- Best diagnostic sign
  - Smooth, tapered ICA narrowing, spares bulb, stops at skull base
  - Similar common carotid artery (CCA), extends superiorly (from aortic arch)
- Secondary occlusion, emboli, stroke are common
CT Findings
- Non-contrast
  - May be negative (vessel often not dilated)
  - +/- Hyperdense carotid space mass (aneurysm from dissection)
- Contrast: May show true, false lumen separated by linear lucency
MR Findings
- Crescentic intramural hematoma on axial images
  - Acute clot iso-, subacute hyperintense on T1-, T2WI
- Eccentrically narrowed residual lumen
  - Possible absent/diminished "flow void," or
  - Slow flow may cause intravascular signal
Other Modality Findings
- Angiography (DSA/CTA/MRA)
  - Smooth/regular tapered narrowing +/- intimal flap
  - May have extraluminal pouch (dissecting aneurysm)
  - May occlude true lumen

Carotid Dissection

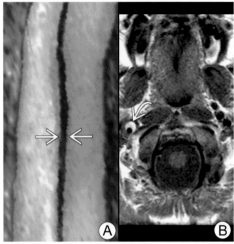

(A) Color Doppler image of common carotid dissection extending from aortic arch. A thick, rigid membrane (arrow) separates two patent lumens. (B) Axial T1WI (level of the nasopharynx) shows a high signal crescent in the wall of right ICA (curved arrow) due to T1 shortening from methemoglobin. This is highly specific.

- Ultrasound
  - Smooth, tapered stenosis or occlusion
    - CCA (from arch): Both lumens usually patent
    - ICA: False lumen occluded, variable patency true lumen
    - Intervening septum: Thick or thin, movable or rigid, depending on wall components included and chronicity

Imaging Recommendations
- US not primary diagnostic tool (dissection may be incidental finding)
- MR (fat-suppressed T1WI helpful for subacute clot), contrast enhanced MRA to define extent and patency
- DSA if MR/MRA negative

Differential Diagnosis
Fibromuscular Dysplasia (FMD)
- "String of beads" appearance > long tubular narrowing
- FMD may cause dissection

Thrombosis
- Often involves bulb
- Intraarterial contrast may delineate intraluminal clot, meniscus

Atherosclerosis
- Involves bulb
- Irregular > smooth tapered narrowing
- Ca++ often present

Vasospasm (Catheter-Induced or Spontaneous)

Pathology
General
- General Path Comments
  - Can occur between or within any layers, subintimal > subadventitial

Carotid Dissection

- o Arch dissections: 15% extend into CCA (usually right, not beyond bulb)
- o ICA dissection
  - Skull base most common
  - 15% multiple, simultaneous cervical dissections (e.g., both ICA, carotid and vertebral)
  - 12% temporal recurrence, rarely same vessel
- Etiology-Pathogenesis
  - o Congenital or acquired defect in internal elastic lamina
  - o Trauma
    - Penetrating or blunt, stretching/torsion (including chiropractic)
    - Minor neck torsion, trivial trauma in 25%: E.g., intense physical activity, coughing, sneezing (is trauma really the cause?)
    - Post endarterectomy (usually with patch graft)
  - o Spontaneous
    - Underlying vasculopathy common (e.g., Marfan, Ehlers-Danlos)
    - Familial ICA dissection may occur
    - Hypertension in 1/3 of all patients
- Epidemiology: Annual incidence of ICA dissection = 3.5 per 100,000

Clinical Issues
Presentation
- CCA dissection
  - o Symptoms due to aortic arch dissection
  - o Uncommon neurological deficit, stroke
- ICA dissection
  - o 70% of patients between 35-50 years old
  - o Male = Female
  - o Headache, neck/facial pain
    - 60-90% of patients with cervical ICA dissection
    - Onset a few hours up to 3-4 weeks
  - o Horner's syndrome in 1/3
  - o Uncommon: Cranial nerve palsy (CN XII > IX, X, XI)
  - o Hemispheric ischemic symptoms may occur
  - o Stroke uncommon, but 45% severe (global MCA)
Natural History
- Usually resolves spontaneously (6-8 weeks)
- Occluded ICA: Frequent spontaneous flow restoration (lysis of thrombus)
Treatment
- Antithrombotics
- Surgery or angioplasty/stent: Aneurysm, high-grade stenosis/symptoms
Prognosis
- No residual or mild neurologic deficit in 70%
- Disabling neurologic deficit in 25%
- Fatal in 5%

Selected References
1. Lee WW et al: Bilateral internal carotid artery dissection due to trivial trauma. J Emerg Med 19: 35-41, 2000
2. Oelerich M et al: Craniocervical artery dissection: MR imaging and MR angiographic findings. Eur Radiol 9: 1385-91, 1999
3. Zielinski T et al: Persistent dissection of carotid artery in patients operated on for type A acute aortic dissection--carotid ultrasound follow-up. Int J Cardiol 70: 133-9, 1999

Vertebral Dissection

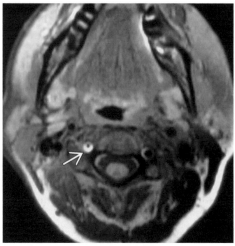

T1W axial image demonstrates crescentic methemoglobin (arrow) in right vertebral artery, indicating dissection. (Courtesy T. Masaryk MD)

Key Facts

- Definition: Hemorrhage into damaged vessel wall with subsequent stenosis or pseudoaneurysm
- Classic imaging appearance: Enlarged external diameter of the artery with intramural crescentic T1 hyperintensity
- Carotid and vertebral dissection responsible for 2% of all cerebrovascular accidents
  - Causes 10-25% of all infarcts in young and middle-aged patients
- Posttraumatic neurological symptoms may be delayed
  - More than one week after the initial injury
- 3D time-of-flight MR angiography
  - Less sensitive for vertebral artery dissection compared to conventional angiography
  - Equally sensitive for carotid artery dissection

Imaging Findings

General Features

- Best imaging clue: T1 hyperintensity surrounding a diminished flow void

MR Findings

- Intramural hematoma
  - Hyperintense on fat suppressed T1WI and T2WI
    - May be isointense initially
  - Crescentic, circumferential, or filling the entire lumen
  - May enhance after intravenous gadolinium
  - May spiral along the artery
- Normal or narrowed flow void
- Thin, curvilinear, hypointense intimal flap
- Subarachnoid hemorrhage may be present if intracranial extension (10%)
- MR angiography
  - Intramural hematoma intermediate signal intensity between flow-related enhancement and surrounding soft tissue

Vertebral Dissection

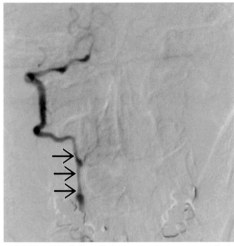

Confirmation of right vertebral dissection as on previous page on catheter angiogram (arrows). (Courtesy T. Masaryk MD)

- May be isointense to soft tissue
o Flow enhancement in pseudoaneurysm

<u>Conventional Angiography Findings</u>
- Most common at C1-2 vertebral bodies
- Smoothly or slightly irregular tapered luminal narrowing
  o Slight stenosis -> "string sign" -> total occlusion
- Pseudoaneurysm (25-35%)
- Intimal flap (10%) and double lumen
- Branch vessel occlusion from embolization

<u>Imaging Recommendations</u>
- Axial T1WI with fat saturation through neck

Differential Diagnosis
<u>Atherosclerotic Disease</u>
- At vertebral artery origin
- More focal
- No intramural hematoma

<u>Fibromuscular Disease</u>
- Can present with focal narrowing on conventional angiogram
- Vertebral artery involvement (7%) less common than carotid (85%)
- No intramural hematoma

Pathology
<u>General</u>
- Genetics
  o Connective tissue disorder predisposing to spontaneous dissection
    - Present in up to 25% of patients with dissection
    - Ehlers-Danlos syndrome, Marfan's syndrome, autosomal dominant polycystic kidney disease
  o Other arteriopathies
    - Fibromuscular dysplasia (15%)

Vertebral Dissection

- Cystic medial necrosis
- Embryology-Anatomy
  - Sites of greater mobility most susceptible to injury
    - Proximal: Between the origin in the subclavian artery to C6 transverse processes
    - Distal: Cranial to C2 transverse processes, before entering the dura
- Etiology-Pathogenesis
  - Spontaneous
  - Hypertension: Primary or drug-induced, including over-the-counter, e.g., ephedrine
  - Major penetrating or blunt trauma
  - Trivial trauma (coughing, sneezing, roller-coaster ride, chiropractic)
    - Prolonged or sudden neck hyperextension or rotation may be a precipitating factor
  - Intimal tear or ruptured vasa vasorum -> intramural hematoma -> stenosis or pseudoaneurysm -> thrombus formation -> emboli
  - Underlying atherosclerosis uncommon
- Epidemiology
  - Estimate of 1 to 1.5 per 100,000
  - Affecting all ages, peak in the fifth decade of life

Microscopic Features
- Hematoma within the tunica media of the vessel wall
  - Compressing the intima, distending the adventitia

Clinical Issues
Presentation
- May affect multiple vessels
  - Horner's syndrome if carotid artery involved
- Unilateral or bilateral occipital headache and posterior neck pain
- Unilateral arm pain or weakness
- Brainstem infarct
  - Lateral medullary syndrome of Wallenberg
- Cerebellar or posterior cerebral artery territory ischemia

Natural History
- Spontaneously healing or recanalization in most cases

Treatment
- Anticoagulation, unless contraindications present
- If persistent ischemia or recurrent embolic events
  - Surgical ligation or endovascular occlusion
  - Percutaneous angioplasty

Prognosis
- Resolution or significant improvement of stenosis in 90% within the first 2 to 3 months
- Recurrence rate of 8%, 50% within the first month

Selected References
1. Schievink WI: Spontaneous dissection of the carotid and vertebral arteries. N Engl J Med 344: 898-906, 2001
2. Provenzale JM: Dissection of the internal carotid and vertebral arteries: Imaging features. AJR 165: 1099-104, 1995
3. Levy C et al: Carotid and vertebral artery dissection: Three-dimensional time-of-flight MR angiography and MR imaging versus conventional angiography. Radiology 190: 97-103, 1994

Aberrant Internal Carotid Artery

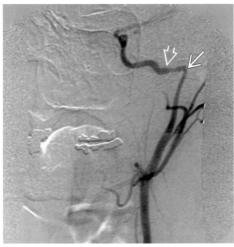

Aberrant internal carotid artery. Left common carotid artery angiogram seen from anterior-posterior perspective shows absence of a normal internal carotid artery. Instead, the enlarged inferior tympanic artery-caroticotympanic artery complex (arrow) is seen anastomosing with the distal internal carotid artery (open arrow).

Key Facts
- Definition: Aberrant internal carotid artery (AbICA) = congenital vascular anomaly resulting from **regression of cervical ICA** during embryogenesis
- Classic imaging appearance: AbICA enters posterior middle ear cavity from below, hugs cochlear promontory as it crosses middle ear, then joins posterior lateral margin of horizontal petrous ICA
- Otoscopic appearance of this vascular-appearing retrotympanic lesion mimics glomus tympanicum & jugulotympanicum paraganglioma
- Radiologist must hold onto correct imaging diagnosis against clinical impression of paraganglioma
- Disaster lurks if misdiagnosis results in biopsy

Imaging Findings
General Features
- Best imaging clue: **Tubular** nature of AbICA
- Tubular lesion crossing middle ear cavity from posterior to anterior
- Absent normal vertical segment of the petrous ICA
CT Findings
- **CT** appearance of AbICA is **diagnostic**
- AbICA enters posterior middle ear through an **enlarged inferior tympanic canaliculus**
- Courses anteriorly across cochlear promontory to join horizontal carotid canal through a dehiscence in carotid plate
- Stenosis at the point where it rejoins horizontal carotid canal sometimes occurs & can lead to pulsatile tinnitus
- **Aberrant stapedial artery** is often associated with AbICA
  - Enlarged anterior tympanic segment of VII
  - Absent foramen spinosum
- Coronal CT shows a round soft-tissue density on cochlear promontory

Aberrant Internal Carotid Artery

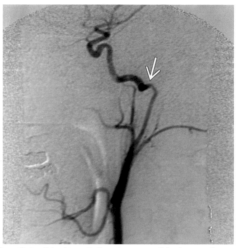

Aberrant internal carotid artery. Left common carotid artery angiogram seen from lateral perspective shows to better advantage enlarged inferior tympanic artery-caroticotympanic artery complex anastomosing with the distal internal carotid artery (arrow). Notice narrowing at this point that may cause pulsatile tinnitus.

- o On a single slice looks disturbingly like paraganglioma
- o Viewing multiple slices reveals tubular nature

MRA & Angiography Findings
- Conventional MR does not reliably identify aberrant ICA
- Lack of MR signal contrast between low signal of mobile proton poor bone and low signal from AbICA blood flow precludes MR diagnosis
- MRA source & reprojected images show aberrant arterial nature of this lesion
    - o Side-to-side comparison shows AbICA enters skull base posterolateral to opposite normal side
    - o On a frontal reprojection, AbICA looks like a 7 (right) or a reverse 7 (left) depending on side of involvement
- Angiography no longer necessary to confirm this imaging diagnosis

Imaging Recommendations
- Bone-only temporal bone CT makes this diagnosis
- If MR done, MRA source and reprojection images are diagnostic

Differential Diagnosis: Vascular Retrotympanic Mass
Dehiscent Jugular Bulb
- Focal absence of sigmoid plate
- Bud from superolateral jugular bulb enters middle ear cavity

Cholesterol Granuloma, Middle Ear
- CT appearance often identical to acquired cholesteatoma
- T1 MR non-contrasted high signal is highly suggestive

Paraganglioma
- Glomus tympanicum
    - o Focal mass on cochlear promontory
    - o No tubular shape
- Glomus jugulotympanicum
    - o Mass enters middle ear through medial floor

Aberrant Internal Carotid Artery

- o CT shows permeative bone changes between jugular foramen & middle ear mass

Aneurysm, Petrous Internal Carotid Artery
- Bone-only CT shows focal smooth expansion of petrous ICA canal
- MRA is diagnostic of aneurysm

Pathology
General
- Embryology-Anatomy
  - o Regression of cervical ICA during embryogenesis triggers a secondary anastomosis to occur between **inferior tympanic artery** and **caroticotympanic artery**
  - o No normal vertical segment of petrous ICA is present
  - o **Inferior tympanic canaliculus** enlarges to accommodate enlarged inferior tympanic artery
  - o Bony margin of posterolateral horizontal petrous ICA canal is dehiscent to allow AbICA to rejoin ICA at this point
- Etiology-Pathogenesis
  - o Occurs when **enlarged inferior tympanic artery** anastomoses with enlarged **caroticotympanic artery** resulting from regression of cervical ICA during embryogenesis
- Epidemiology
  - o Very rare vascular anomaly
  - o At least 30% have aberrant stapedial artery associated

Clinical Issues
Presentation
- Principal presenting symptom: Vascular retrotympanic mass
- Other symptoms
  - o Objective or subjective pulsatile tinnitus (PT)
    - Objective PT when stenosis is present at junction of AbICA & normal horizontal petrous ICA
  - o Conductive hearing loss
- Otoscopic exam: **Vascular retrotympanic mass** behind inferior TM
- Important clinical observation: Vascular-appearing retrotympanic mass may exactly mimic paraganglioma

Treatment
- Most patients have minor symptoms that do not require treatment
- A clinical-radiologic mistake in diagnosis with resultant surgical intervention can be disastrous & must be avoided at all cost!

Prognosis
- No long term sequelae reported with AbICA
- Poor prognosis results only if misdiagnosis leads to biopsy
- If PT is loud, can be debilitating

Selected References
1. Botma M et al: Aberrant internal carotid artery in the middle-ear space. J Laryngol Otol 114: 784-7, 2000
2. Davis WL et al: MR angiography of an aberrant internal carotid artery. AJNR 12: 1225, 1991
3. Lo WW et al: Aberrant carotid artery: Radiologic diagnosis with emphasis in high-resolution computed tomography. RadioGraphics 5: 985-93, 1985

Persistent Stapedial Artery

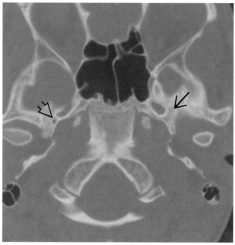

Persistent stapedial artery. Axial CT through the skull base in this patient with left persistent stapedial artery shows the characteristic absent foramen spinosum (arrow) ipsilateral to the lesion. The normal foramen spinosum is seen on the right (open arrow) just posterolateral to the foramen ovale.

Key Facts
- Definition: Rare congenital vascular anomaly in which embryological stapedial artery persists resulting in an aberrant vascular pathway
- Classic imaging appearance
  - NECT: **Absent foramen spinosum** & subtle enlargement of anterior tympanic segment of facial nerve canal on ipsilateral side
- Other key facts
  - May be **associated with aberrant internal carotid artery** (AbICA)
  - Majority **asymptomatic**, found incidentally at surgery or on radiological workup
  - Rarely presents with tinnitus &/or pulsatile retrotympanic red mass

Imaging Findings
General Features
- Best imaging clue
  - CT shows persistent stapedial artery (PSA) as absent foramen spinosum & **subtle** enlargement of anterior tympanic facial nerve canal
CT Findings
- Absent foramen spinosum on ipsilateral side
- Subtle enlargement of facial nerve canal or separate canal parallel to normal facial nerve canal
- Curvilinear structure crossing medial wall of middle ear cavity over cochlear promontory
- Small canaliculus leaving carotid canal
MR Findings
- Conventional MR shows nothing
- MRA may show absent middle meningeal artery
Cerebral Angiography Findings
- External carotid arteriogram
  - Shows absence of normal middle meningeal artery

Persistent Stapedial Artery

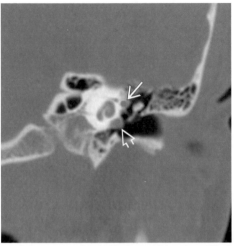

Persistent stapedial artery associated with aberrant internal carotid artery. Coronal CT of left temporal bone shows the persistent stapedial artery as an enlarged anterior tympanic segment of the facial nerve canal (arrow). Aberrant internal carotid artery is seen on the cochlear promontory (open arrow).

- Internal Carotid Arteriogram
  - Shows PSA arising from intrapetrosal portion of ICA or from an AbICA

Imaging Recommendations
- Thin section, NECT through temporal bone in axial & coronal planes
  - Facial nerve tumor involving the anterior aspect of tympanic segment can be excluded
  - Knowledge of pathogenesis of pulsatile mass may prevent unnecessary surgery, or help in surgical planning

Differential Diagnosis: Abnormal Intratemporal Facial Nerve

Bell's Herpetic Facial Neuritis
- CT normal
- T1 C+ shows entire intratemporal facial nerve enhances

Facial Nerve Hemangioma
- CT commonly shows intratumoral ossification
- T1 C+ MR shows irregular enhancing mass in geniculate fossa

Facial Nerve Schwannoma
- CT shows tubular or focal enlargement of facial nerve canal
- T1 C+ shows mass enhancing

Pathology

General
- General Path Comments
  - Congenital anomaly
  - Often seen with AbICA
- Genetics
  - Other associations reported include
    - Trisomy 13, 15, and 21
    - Paget's disease

Persistent Stapedial Artery

- Otosclerosis
- Anencephaly
- Neurofibromatosis
- Embryology-Anatomy
  - Primitive 2nd aortic arch gives rise to hyoid artery
  - Hyoid artery gives rise to stapedial artery
  - Stapedial artery divides into dorsal (middle meningeal artery) & ventral divisions (to maxilla & mandible)
    - PSA courses from infracochlear carotid through stapedial obturator foramen
    - It enlarges tympanic facial nerve canal on its way to middle cranial fossa to become the middle meningeal artery
- Etiology-Pathogenesis
  - Stapedial artery fails to involute in third fetal month
  - As a result the developing vasculature changes course
- Epidemiology
  - Prevalence = 0.48%

Clinical Issues
Presentation
- Most common symptom or sign: Asymptomatic finding at surgery or on temporal bone CT
- If symptomatic, pulsatile tinnitus
- Otoscopic exam
  - Most commonly normal
  - Rarely a pulsatile, red, retrotympanic mass is seen
- Surgical implications
  - PSA can complicate stapedectomy or cholesteatoma resection
  - PSA may prevent cochlear implantation
Treatment
- Generally left alone if asymptomatic and incidental
- If presumed cause of pulsatile tinnitus, surgical ligation or endovascular occlusion may be considered
  - Only done if pulsatile tinnitus is intractable
Prognosis
- Excellent if left alone

Selected References
1. Tien et al: Persistent stapedial artery. Otol Neurotol 22: 975-6, 2001
2. Thiers et al: Persistent stapedial artery: CT findings. AJNR 21: 1551-4, 2000
3. Silbergleit et al: Persistent stapedial artery. AJNR 21: 572-7, 2000

Hemangioma of the Head and Neck

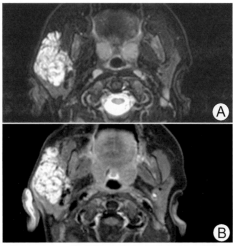

Parotid space hemangioma. (A) Axial T2WI demonstrates a well-defined, lobulated mass within the parotid space, with sharp margins, and mild surrounding mass effect. (B) Axial T1WI C+ demonstrates corresponding enhancement of the mass.

Key Facts
- Synonyms: Capillary/cavernous hemangioma, infantile/congenital/juvenile hemangioma, benign hemangioendothelioma
- Definition: Rare, benign congenital neoplasm composed of proliferating endothelial cells (c.f. vascular/lymphatic malformations, do not have increased endothelial turnover)
- Classic imaging appearance: Lobulated, enhancing mass, with little surrounding mass effect
- Classically divided into capillary (70%), cavernous, and mixed types
- Found within soft tissues, intraosseous, or intramuscular (rare)
- Most common head and neck tumor of infancy
  - Parotid hemangioma most common salivary neoplasm in children
- Cavernous hemangioma (CavH) most common orbital tumor in adults
- Laryngeal hemangiomas more common in adults, but more likely to cause airway obstruction in pediatric cases

Imaging Findings
General Features
- Best imaging clue: Enhancing, lobulated, solid mass with mild mass effect
- CavH is sharply marginated; capillary type (CapH) may be poorly defined
CT Findings
- NECT: iso- or slightly hyperdense (possible microcalcifications), well-defined mass may extend superficially to skin
- May have benign remodeling of surrounding osseous structures
- CECT: Avid homogeneous enhancement
MR Findings
- T1WI: Low - intermediate heterogeneous SI, diffuse intense enhancement
  - May see flow voids from vessels/sinusoids within lesion
  - May see high signal intensity from fatty replacement within lesion
- T2WI: Usually high signal intensity

Hemangioma of the Head and Neck

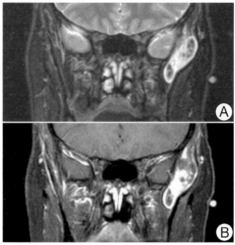

Intramuscular hemangioma. (A) Coronal T2WI demonstrates a well-defined mass within the left masticator space with extension into the suprazygomatic masticator space. (B) Coronal T1WI C+ shows correlating enhancement within the mass, with mild mass effect, and no surrounding aggressive changes.

- Prior hemorrhage/slow flow may cause foci of high T1 and T2 SI
- CavH usually has hypointense rim (pseudocapsule)

Other Modality Findings
- Plain film views may show phleboliths to suggest the diagnoses (15%)
- US demonstrates well-defined hypoechoic mass with heterogeneous echotexture, cystic spaces, occasional phleboliths
  - o Color Doppler demonstrates flow signal, with low resistance

Imaging Recommendations
- MRI useful for lesion location and relationship to vital structures
- CavH may show initial central enhancement with later filling-in on dynamic contrasted CT and MRI studies

Differential Diagnosis: Pediatric Transpatial Head and Neck Mass

Cystic Hygroma
- Fluid-filled, well-defined, loculated, insinuating cystic mass
- Congenital malformation of lymphatic channels

Epidermoid/Dermoid
- Slowly growing, unilocular, nonenhancing mass
- Epidermoid – lined with simple squamous epithelium, with fluid density/intensity
- Dermoid – epithelial lining with skin appendages, mixed/fat density/intensity

Abscess
- Presenting symptoms depend on location
- Fluid collection with septations and enhancing, thick, irregular wall

Pathology

General
- General Path Comments

Hemangioma of the Head and Neck

  o Pathological differences between CapH and CavH, may be multiple
- Etiology-Pathogenesis
  o Dilation of vascular spaces, marked endothelial mitotic activity
- Epidemiology
  o More common in white infants; female > male (3:1)
  o 50% of all CapH occur in the head and neck
  o 5% of all salivary gland tumors
  o 2% incidence in neonates, more common in preterm infants
  o 10% incidence by 1yo

Gross Pathologic or Surgical Features
- Discrete, reddish vascular mass
- CapH - may have significant blood supply from internal and external carotid arteries, therefore extensive bleeding may occur
- CavH – surrounding pseudocapsule of compressed surrounding tissue, without significant arterial supply

Microscopic Features
- CapH – unencapsulated small vascular spaces lined by benign endothelial cells with capillary and endothelial vessel proliferation
  o May be positive for immunochemical factor VIII staining
- CavH – encapsulated large vascular channels lined with thin, attenuated epithelial cells

Clinical Issues

Presentation
- Presentation depends on location; unilateral facial swelling, possibly with an underlying vascular hue in a child, that may blanch with pressure
- Soft, compressible mass may increase in size with crying of child (50%)

Natural History
- Rare systemic complications: Cardiac failure, Kasabach-Merritt syndrome (triad of hemangioma, thrombocytopenia, and coagulopathy)
- CapH will usually increase in size for 6-10 months, then slowly regress
  o Predominant type in first year of life – tumor of infants
- May rapidly increase in size; undergo fatty replacement by adolescence

Treatment
- Treatment based on location and extent of tumor
- Many lesions will spontaneous regress (50% by 5yo, 70% by 7yo), therefore surgery is often postponed until adulthood unless symptomatic
- Steroid/interferon therapy, laser surgery, intravascular embolization for non-intraorbital lesions
- CavH of the orbit often easily excised due to pseudocapsule
- CapH very responsive to steroid therapy, usually spontaneously regress
- Angiography with possible embolization may assist prior to surgery

Prognosis
- Excellent prognosis with complete excision
- Recurrence rates: CapH: 20%, CavH: 9%, mixed: 28%
- May have high complication rates if insinuating vital structures

Selected References
1. Makeieff M et al: Intramuscular hemangioma of posterior neck muscles. Eur Arch Otorhinolaryngol 258(1): 28-30, 2001
2. Robertson RL et al: Head and neck vascular anomalies of childhood. Neuroimaging Clin of N Amer 9(1): 115-31, 1999
3. Yang WT et al: Sonographic features of head and neck hemangiomas and vascular malformations: review of 23 patients. J Ultrasound Med 16(1): 39-44, 1997

Dehiscent Jugular Bulb

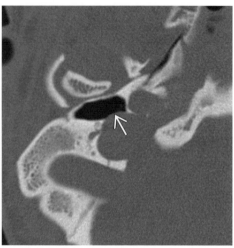

Dehiscent jugular bulb. Axial CT through the right temporal bone at the level of the low EAC shows a broad defect in the sigmoid plate (arrow). The dehiscent jugular bulb protrudes into the hypotympanum through this bony defect.

Key Facts
- Synonyms: Exposed jugular bulb (JB), jugular megabulb deformity, lateral JB diverticulum
- Definition: Normal venous variant where there is superior & lateral extension of JB into middle ear cavity through a dehiscent sigmoid plate
- Classic imaging appearance: CT shows a soft-tissue mass contiguous with JB projecting into the middle ear cavity through a dehiscent sigmoid plate
- Other key facts
  - Dehiscent jugular bulb (DJB) more commonly seen with high-riding JB
  - High-riding JB is more commonly present on right

Imaging Findings
General Features
- Best imaging clue
  - Focal dehiscence of sigmoid plate with protruding mass extending into posteroinferior middle ear cavity seen on CT
CT Findings
- NECT: Soft tissue mass in middle ear cavity inseparable from JB
  - **Sigmoid plate** is **dehiscent**
  - DJB projects into posteroinferior aspect of middle ear cavity
- CECT: Protruding mass enhances to same degree as JB
MR Findings
- Turbulent venous flow may make JB difficult to evaluate by MR
- Coronal images show lateral lobulation-projection of JB into inferior middle ear cavity
- CE T1: Avidly enhancing middle ear mass connects to enhancing JB
- T2: May have heterogeneous iso- to hyperintensity, or flow void
- MRV: JB extends superolaterally into middle ear cavity
- Dynamic MRI: Normal jugular bulb demonstrates a decrease in the dynamic curve at ~ 30 seconds following contrast administration

Dehiscent Jugular Bulb

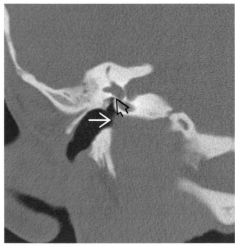

Dehiscent jugular bulb. Coronal CT of the right temporal bone shows the dehiscent jugular bulb (arrow) protruding superolaterally into the middle ear cavity. Also notice the oval window atresia (open arrow).

Venography Findings
- Venography shows "pseudopod" extending off superolateral margin of JB
- Bony landmarks difficult to ascertain

Imaging Recommendations
- Temporal bone CT is best, most diagnostic test
- CE MR with MRV useful in equivocal cases

Differential Diagnosis: Jugular Bulb Mass

Asymmetrically Large JB
- Common normal variant, right prominence more common
- Usually only problem when found incidentally in pulsatile tinnitus workup
- CT of BOS demonstrates intact jugular spine & JB cortical margins

High-Riding JB
- JB cortical margins intact
- Defined by most cephalad portion extending superior to floor of IAC
- Increased signal from complex flow may be present on some MR sequences

JB Diverticulum
- Focal polypoid mass extending from cephalad JB
- Sigmoid plate is intact

Jugulotympanicum Paraganglioma
- CT: Permeative bony changes along JB superolateral margins
- T1WI: Jugular foramen mass with high velocity flow voids ("pepper")
- Vector of spread: Superolateral from JB to floor of middle ear cavity hypotympanum

Jugular Foramen Meningioma
- CT: Permeative-sclerotic bony changes along JB margins
- T1WI: No high velocity flow voids
- CE T1: Dural tails along margins of avidly enhancing mass
- Vector of spread: Centrifugal along dural surfaces

Dehiscent Jugular Bulb

Jugular Foramen Schwannoma
- CT: Smoothly scalloped, enlarged jugular foramen
- CE T1: Dumbbell-shaped enhancing mass in jugular foramen
- Vector of spread: Extend along expected course of cranial nerves 9-11

Pathology
General
- General Path Comments
  - Size of dehiscence dependent on size of sigmoid plate defect
- Embryology-Anatomy: Focal dehiscence in sigmoid plate that normally separates JB from hypotympanum
- Etiology-Pathogenesis
  - Congenital lesion
  - Dehiscence more commonly seen with high-riding jugular bulb
- Epidemiology: 7% of cadaveric cases
Gross Pathologic or Surgical Features
- Vascular "mass" seen in posterior & inferior middle ear cavity, inseparable from jugular bulb

Clinical Issues
Presentation
- Most common presenting symptom: **Asymptomatic**
- Other presenting symptoms
  - DJB has been reported linked to many symptoms
  - Debate as to whether it is causal of any symptom complex
  - Pulsatile tinnitus, headache, hearing loss all have be linked to DJB
  - Conductive hearing loss secondary to
    - Obstruction of round window by DJB
    - DJB impinges on tympanic membrane
    - DJB impinges on ossicular chain
    - Combination of above
- Otoscopic exam
  - Vascular-blue "mass" behind an intact TM
  - Seen in posterior-inferior TM quadrant
  - Valsalva or ipsilateral jugular venous compression often shows distention of mass on otologic exam
Natural History
- Congenital lesion that does **not** grow with time
Treatment
- Initial therapy: Treatment should rarely be employed
- Surgical correction
  - Surgical reconstruction with wax interposition or septal cartilage homograft placed over sigmoid plate dehiscence
Prognosis
- Excellent if left alone
- Important radiologic diagnosis to make so injury from myringotomy does not occur

Selected References
1. Marshot-Dupuch K: Pulsatile and nonpulsatile tinnitus: a systematic approach. Seminars in US, CT, and MRI 22: 250-70, 2001
2. Weiss RL et al: High jugular bulb and conductive hearing loss. Laryngoscope, 107, 321-7, 1997
3. Wadin K et al: Effects of a high jugular fossa and jugular bulb diverticulum on the inner ear. Acta Radiol Diagn 27: 629-36, 1986

Jugular Bulb Diverticulum

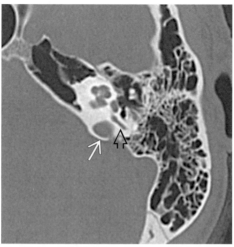

Jugular bulb diverticulum. Axial CT image reveals a cephalad-projecting jugular bulb diverticulum (arrow) posterior to the internal auditory canal and medial to the posterior semicircular canal (open arrow). The bony margin of this lesion is well corticated. The axial image shows only the cephalad tip of the lesion.

Key Facts
- Synonyms: Jugular diverticulum, petrous jugular malposition
- Definition: Congenital vascular anomaly of jugular bulb, with focal "finger-like" projection extending from jugular bulb into surrounding skull base
- Classic imaging appearance
  - Jugular bulb diverticulum (JBD) is seen as a focal polypoid projection extending off margin of jugular bulb
  - Jugular bulb may be high or normal in position
- Other key facts
  - Clinical presentation: Asymptomatic, incidental
  - Normal otologic examination
    - Tympanic membrane (TM) normal
    - Consequently, JBD is a radiologic diagnosis

Imaging Findings
General Features
- Best imaging clue
  - Focal polypoid extension off jugular bulb superiorly into deep temporal bone just behind internal auditory canal (IAC)
- JBD most commonly extends superiorly
  - Other directions of extension include
    - Medial, anterior or posterior
    - When lateral = dehiscent jugular bulb
CT Findings
- NECT: Well-corticated polypoid extension off margin of jugular bulb
- CECT: Uniform enhancement of bulb & JBD
- Radiologist must inspect for local extension
  - Erosion through wall of IAC
    - Important when seen in conjunction with acoustic schwannoma

Jugular Bulb Diverticulum

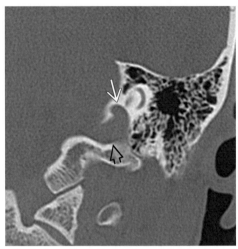

Jugular bulb diverticulum. Coronal temporal bone CT at the level of the mastoid sinuses shows the jugular bulb diverticulum (arrow) as a "finger-like" profection pointed cephalad off the posterior roof of the jugular bulb (open arrow). Again notice the intact cortical margin of this lesion.

MR Findings
- Turbulent flow makes jugular bulb & JBD difficult to evaluate by MR
  - May mimic thrombosis or schwannoma
- CEMR: Avid enhancement may mimic schwannoma
- T2MR: May have heterogeneous high intensity
- MR Venogram (MRV): "Finger-like" projection off jugular bulb
- Dynamic MR: Normal jugular bulb & diverticulum show decrease in dynamic curve at ~ 30 seconds following contrast administration

Imaging Recommendations
- Start with non-contrasted bone algorithm CT in axial & coronal planes
- If concern lingers, MR with contrast & MRV

Differential Diagnosis: Jugular Bulb Lesion

Asymmetric Large Jugular Bulb
- Common normal variant, right prominence more common
- Usually only problem when found incidentally in skull base work-up
- CT: Intact jugular spine & jugular bulb cortical margins

High-Riding Jugular Bulb
- Defined by most cephalad portion extending superior to floor of IAC
- CT: Jugular foramen cortical margins intact
- MR: Complex or increased signal does not persist on all MR sequences

Dehiscent Jugular Bulb
- Vascular retrotympanic mass
- CT: Sigmoid plate shows focal dehiscence

Jugulotympanicum Paraganglioma
- Enhancing mass in jugular foramen
- CT: Permeative bony changes on jugular foramen margins
- T1WI: High velocity flow voids ("pepper")

Jugular Bulb Diverticulum

Jugular Foramen Schwannoma
- Dumbbell-shaped mass following cranial nerves 9-11 course
- NECT: Smoothly scalloped bony margins of enlarged jugular foramen
- T1 CE MR: Fusiform enhancing mass in jugular foramen

Jugular Foramen Meningioma
- Mass in jugular foramen spreading along dural planes
- CT: Permeative-sclerotic jugular foramen bony margins
- CE T1 MR: Dural tails

Pathology
General
- General Path Comments
  - JBD thought to represent expansion of high jugular bulb into surrounding anatomic landscape, but hindered by dense otic capsule
- Embryology-Anatomy
  - High-riding jugular bulb is more commonly seen with poorly aerated mastoid & perilymphatic structures
- Etiology-Pathogenesis
  - JBD may be secondary to hemodynamic factors
  - JBD more commonly seen with high-riding jugular bulb
- Epidemiology
  - Present in 8% of pathologic temporal bone specimens studies
  - Present in 35% of cases with high-riding jugular bulb

Gross Pathologic or Surgical Features
- JBD most commonly extends superiorly & medially, into region between IAC, posterior cranial fossa, and bony vestibular aqueduct

Clinical Issues
Presentation
- Most common symptom or sign: **Asymptomatic**
- Many symptoms have been linked to JBD
  - Based on direction of extension of diverticulum
    - Sensorineural hearing loss thought to be secondary to encroachment of IAC or endolymphatic duct
    - Tinnitus (continuous or intermittent ringing)
    - Vertigo
    - Symptoms mimicking Ménière's disease
- Symptoms reported to have a tenuous link to JBD

Natural History
- Congenital lesion fixed early in life

Treatment
- Conservative management of symptoms
- Surgical intervention no longer recommended

Selected References
1. Kobanawa S et al: Jugular bulb diverticulum associated with lower cranial nerve palsy and multiple aneurysms. Surg Neurol 53(6): 559-62, 2000
2. Atilla S et al: Computed tomographic evaluation of surgically significant vascular variations related with the temporal bone. Eur J Radiol 20(1): 52-6, 1995
3. Wadin K et al: The jugular diverticulum a radioanatomic investigation. Acta Radiol Diagn 27(4): 395-401, 1986

Carotid Pseudoaneurysm, Extracranial

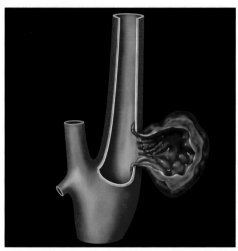

Graphic illustration depicts traumatic pseudoaneurysm of the cervical internal carotid artery. Complete disruption of the ICA wall has resulted in a paravascular hematoma. Hematoma cavitation can create a patent channel with the parent vessel. Pseudoaneurysms do not contain components of the normal vessel wall.

Key Facts
- Synonym: "False" aneurysm
- Definition: Paravascular cavitated clot in continuity with cervical internal carotid artery (ICA)
- Classic imaging appearance: Carotid space (CS) mass that communicates directly with carotid artery
- Usually occurs with trauma (blunt or penetrating)
- Pseudoaneurysms do not contain layers of normal vessel wall
- > 80% of all cervical vascular injuries involve carotid arteries

Imaging Findings
General Features
- Best imaging clue: Contrast extravasation into extraluminal, paravascular cavity
CT Findings
- NECT
  - Round/ovoid/lobulated isodense mass in CS
- CECT
  - Irregular widening of vessel contour
  - Outpouching of contrast from ICA
  - May compress true ICA lumen
MR Findings
- T1WI: Inhomogeneous (usually isointense +/- flow void, phase artifact)
- T2WI: Inhomogeneous (mixed hypo/hyperintense +/- flow void)
Other Modality Findings
- Angiography (DSA/CTA): Findings vary from small saccular to fusiform dilatations, large cavitating hematoma
- Color Doppler U/S: Turbulent flow in lesion with high peripheral resistance vascular bed

Carotid Pseudoaneurysm, Extracranial

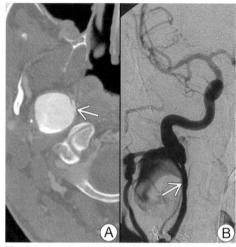

A 31-year-old male had vocal cord paralysis after a motor vehicle accident. (A) CECT scan shows a vascular carotid space mass that communicates directly with the compressed ICA (arrow). (B) DSA shows a large pseudoaneurysm opacified with a jet of contrast. Note ICA compression, displacement (arrow).

Imaging Recommendations
- Duplex sonography good rapid screening examination in acute setting of suspected cervical vascular injury
- CECT + CTA
- DSA if penetrating injury in surgical zone I (below sternal notch) or III (angle of mandible to skull base)

Differential Diagnosis
Dissecting Aneurysm
- Intramural hematoma dilates vessel wall, ruptures through intima
- False lumen establishes continuity with true lumen
Arteriovenous Fistula
- May occur as rare complication of pseudoaneurysm
- Carotid pseudoaneurysm ruptures, establishes continuity with internal and/or external jugular vein, branches
- Contrast injected into common carotid artery (CCA) fills pseudoaneurysm, rapidly opacifies internal jugular vein (IJV)

Pathology
General
- General Path Comments
  - "True" aneurysm contains layers of normal vessel wall; "false" or pseudoaneurysm does not
- Etiology-Pathogenesis
  - Partial/complete vessel wall disruption results in periluminal hemorrhage
  - Paravascular clot forms, cavitates, communicates with parent vessel
- Epidemiology
  - 1/3 of cervical ICA vascular injuries caused by penetrating trauma

Carotid Pseudoaneurysm, Extracranial

Gross Pathologic or Surgical Features
- Bluish-purple paravascular CS mass contained by fascia and/or adventitia

Microscopic Features
- Wall of pseudoaneurysm is organized hematoma
- Does not contain intima, internal elastic lamina, muscularis; may be contained by adventitia

Clinical Issues

Presentation
- Can be occult, asymptomatic (2.5% of patients with blunt injury)
- 50-60% have palpable cervical mass (+/- pulsation)
- 40% neurologic symptoms
  - Horner syndrome
  - CN IX-XI palsy
  - Cerebral ischemia/infarction
- Rare: Carotid rupture ("blow out")

Natural History
- Variable; may enlarge, resolve spontaneously, undergo thrombosis

Treatment
- Goal: Occlusion of pseudoaneurysm with preservation of ICA
- Can be surgical or interventional

Prognosis
- No reliable findings to prognosticate whether lesions will improve
- 45% combined stroke/mortality rate after ligation of parent vessel
- 23% stroke/mortality with observation only
- 10% if parent vessel repaired, reconstructed

Selected References
1. Guyot LL et al: Vascular injury in neurotrauma. Neurol Res 23: 291-6, 2001
2. LeBlang SD et al: Noninvasive imaging of cervical vascular injuries. AJR 174: 1269-78, 2000
3. Munera F et al: Diagnosis of arterial injuries caused by penetrating trauma to the neck. Radiol 216: 356-62, 2000

Arteriovenous Fistula in the Neck

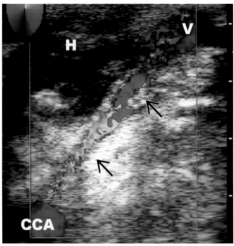

Carotid artery AVF following attempted jugular vein cannulation. Turbulent flow is seen in a fistulous communication (arrows) between the common carotid artery (CCA) and an unnamed superficial vein (V). US examination followed the development of ecchymosis and a soft-tissue hematoma (H).

Key Facts
- Acronym: AVF
- Definition: Fistulous communication between a neck artery and vein, trauma-related or iatrogenic
- Classic imaging appearance
  - CTA, MRA, DSA: Tract between artery and vein, with contrast opacification of draining vein during arterial phase
  - Ultrasound (US): Tract between artery and vein, with high velocity, turbulent/pulsatile venous flow
- Other key facts
  - Most frequent between carotid artery and internal jugular vein, less common vertebral
  - Vascular trauma much more frequent with penetrating injury (36%) than contusion (1%)
  - Iatrogenic injury (venous access) is common cause

Imaging Findings
General Features
- Best imaging clue
  - Imaging shows artery-vein connection
CT Findings
- Contrast enhancement required, multidetector CTA state of art
- Arteriovenous communication (broad or narrow, short or long) on CTA
- Early filling (appearance) of draining vein
- Hematoma/soft tissue edema in area of injury
- Possible pseudoaneurysm accompanying fistula
- Possible additional arterial injury (intimal flap, dissection, stenosis, occlusion)
- Possible hyperdynamic circulation

Arteriovenous Fistula in the Neck

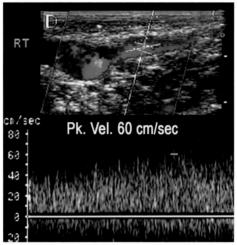

AVF draining vein. High velocity flow is seen in the superficial vein draining the carotid AVF. Peak velocity is 60 cm/sec, a value normally seen in arteries.

MR Findings
- Analogous to CT
- AVF may be identified using TOF/phase contrast MRA, but turbulence induced artifacts may be confusing
- 3D MRA with contrast enhancement preferred (state of art)
- MRA may be cumbersome to perform in acute trauma setting

Ultrasound Findings
- High velocity, turbulent flow in draining vein, may also be pulsatile
- Marked turbulence in fistula
- Possible soft-tissue vibrations on color Doppler (montage of color in soft tissues)
- High velocity, low resistance flow pattern in feeding artery
- Other findings analogous to CT

Imaging Recommendations
- DSA (and radiographic intervention) or surgery for acute, life threatening cervical vascular emergencies
- Vascular injury uncertain, acute but patient stable: CTA assessment
  - Quick and accurate method for vascular evaluation
  - Defines scope of soft-tissue injury, size of hematoma
  - Identifies concomitant bone or airway injury
- Vascular injury uncertain, subacute trauma
  - MRA or CTA: Preferred, comprehensive evaluation from arch to head
  - Color Doppler US: Cost effective, accurate, convenient (bedside), but limited field of view
- Note: Unrecognized vascular injury, although uncommon, can lead to significant complications; it is argued that all patients with substantial cervical soft-tissue injury (including contusion) should be evaluated for occult vascular damage

Arteriovenous Fistula in the Neck

Differential Diagnosis
Arteriovenous Malformation
- Early venous drainage, as in AVF
- "Tangle" of veins connecting artery and draining vein

Vascular Injury or Compression
- May produce audible bruit, turbulence on US
- No early venous drainage or other AVF findings

Pseudoaneurysm
- May produce audible bruit
- Readily diagnosed with all imaging modalities

Pathology
General
- General Path Comments
  - AVF most common with penetrating injury, but can occur with contusion
  - AVF commonly involves carotid artery, but can involve vertebral or other cervical arteries
- Etiology-Pathogenesis
  - Laceration of artery and vein with establishment of a soft-tissue fistulous communication
  - Mycotic aneurysm with tissue destruction extending to adjacent vein

Clinical Issues
Presentation
- Acute
  - Visible open neck trauma
  - Neck contusion/hematoma (possibly expanding)
  - Iatrogenic, post-procedural hematoma
  - Audible bruit, palpable thrill
  - Dilated, hyperdynamic draining vein
- Subacute, chronic
  - Audible bruit, palpable thrill
  - Dilated, hyperdynamic draining vein
  - Possible delayed rupture of artery
  - Possible high output heart failure
  - Possible cerebral ischemia from "steal" phenomenon

Treatment
- Acute distress, unstable – radiologic intervention or surgical exploration
- Acute but stable, or subacute
  - Radiologic intervention is method of choice
    - Intraarterial stent graft
    - Embolization of artery/vein, if sacrifice of vessel is acceptable
  - Surgical repair

Prognosis
- Excellent with treatment

Selected References
1. Feliciano DV: Management of penetrating injuries to carotid artery. World J Surg 25: 1028-35, 2001
2. LeBlang SD et al: Noninvasive imaging of cervical vascular injuries. AJR 174: 1269-78, 2000
3. Múnera F et al: Diagnosis of arterial injuries caused by penetrating trauma to the neck: Comparison of helical CT angiography and conventional angiography. Radiology 216: 356-62, 2000

Petrous ICA Aneurysm

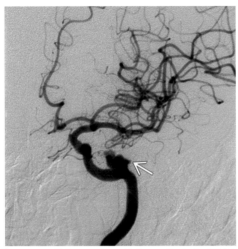

Petrous ICA aneurysm. Oblique angiographic image of selective left internal carotid artery shows an irregular ovoid aneurysm (arrow) projecting cephalad from the proximal portion of the horizontal petrous internal carotid artery. The aneurysm has a broad neck.

Key Facts
- Synonyms: Petrous carotid aneurysm, aneurysm of intrapetrous internal carotid artery
- Definition: Congenital or acquired aneurysm of petrous internal carotid artery; may be found anywhere from its entrance into skull base to its exit into cavernous sinus
- Classic imaging appearance
  - CT: Focal remodeling-enlargement of petrous ICA canal
  - MR: Complex signal, oval to fusiform mass of petrous ICA
- Other key facts
  - Rare vascular lesion in this rigid osseous conduit = petrous ICA canal
  - Devastating consequences if not recognized pre-operatively
  - Treated with endovascular trapping of petrous ICA

Imaging Findings
General Features
- Best imaging clue
  - CT shows expansile lesion of petrous ICA canal
  - MR reveals complex signal mass along petrous ICA
- Most are fusiform (congenital) with intraluminal thrombus
- When focal, posttraumatic or atherosclerotic
CT Findings
- NECT: Focal or fusiform enlargement of petrous ICA canal
  - Curvilinear calcifications in aneurysm wall
- CECT: Enhancing lesion within enlarged petrous ICA canal
MR Findings
- NEMR (T1): Round or fusiform mass with complex signal within lumen
  - Multiple ages of intraluminal clot & flow phenomenon
- MRA: Enlarged, irregular area along petrous ICA

Petrous ICA Aneurysm

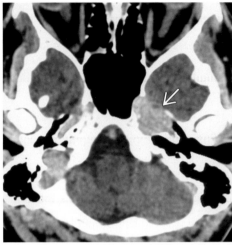

Petrous internal carotid aneurysm. Axial enhanced CT through the skull base reveals an enhancing "mass" (arrow) enlarging the distal horizontal petrous ICA canal. Previous history of significant trauma to the skull base was present in this patient.

- o May be smaller than actual aneurysm since only lumen area with flowing blood is seen

Angiography Findings
- Aneursymal dilatation of petrous ICA
- Size of aneurysm as seen on angiographic image often much smaller than actual aneurysm because of intraluminal clot

Imaging Recommendations
- MR with MRA is best 1ˢᵗ study as it best delineates size, shape & site of aneurysm; absence or presence and extent of intraluminal hemorrhage; patency of petrous ICA
- Thin-section bone only CT confirms location along carotid canal
- Angiography for endovascular therapy, not diagnosis

Differential Diagnosis: Vascular Lesion of Temporal Bone
Aberrant Internal Carotid Artery
- CT shows tubular mass crosses middle ear cavity to rejoin horizontal petrous ICA; large inferior tympanic canaliculus
- Otoscopy: Anteroinferior pulsatile red retrotympanic lesion

Dehiscent Jugular Bulb
- Focal absence of sigmoid plate connects jugular bulb to middle ear "mass"
- Otoscopy: Posteroinferior deep blue retrotympanic lesion

Persistent Stapedial Artery (PSA)
- CT shows subtle enlargement of anterior tympanic segment facial nerve
- CT shows absence of foramen spinosum on side of PSA
- Otoscopy: Normal or subtle pink retrotympanic lesion

Glomus Tympanicum Paraganglioma
- CT shows focal mass on cochlear promontory; not tubular
- T1 C+ MR reveals mass enhances
- Otoscopy: Cherry red pulsatile anteroinferior retrotympanic mass

Glomus Jugulotympanicum Paraganglioma
- CT shows permeative-destructive bony changes on superolateral margin of jugular foramen
- T1 C+ MR reveals enhancing mass extending up from jugular foramen into middle ear cavity
- Otoscopy: Vascular retrotympanic mass that cannot be distinguished from glomus tympanicum paraganglioma

Pathology
General
- Etiology-Pathogenesis
  o Congenital aneurysm most common
  o Posttraumatic pseudoaneurysm less common
  o Atherosclerotic aneurysm least common
- Epidemiology
  o Very rare lesion makes errors in diagnosis common

Gross Pathologic or Surgical Features
- Focal or diffusely enlarged petrous ICA with intraluminal clot

Microscopic Features
- Wall lacks elastic lamina, smooth muscle layers

Clinical Issues
Presentation
- Most common sign/symptom: Hearing loss
- Other signs & symptoms depend on direction of expansion
  o Lateral expansion
    ▪ Vascular retrotympanic mass
    ▪ Conductive hearing loss
    ▪ Otorrhagia &/or epistaxis (blood down eustachian tube)
  o Medial expansion (cavernous sinus)
    ▪ Diplopia
    ▪ 6th nerve palsy
    ▪ Horner's syndrome
- Medical history
  o May have history of skull base fracture

Natural History & Prognosis
- Gradual enlargement
- Distal emboli may occur
- Embolic or occlusive stroke possible if left alone

Treatment
- Endovascular therapy
  o Balloon trapping or aneurysmal obliteration with ICA preservation
  o Endovascular stent placement
- Surgical therapy no longer preferred 1st approach

Selected References
1. Eliason JL et al: Skull base resection with cervical-to-petrous carotid artery bypass to facilitate repair of distal internal carotid artery lesions. Cardiovasc Surg 10: 31-7, 2002
2. Redekop G et al: Treatment of traumatic aneurysmal and arteriovenous fistulas of the skull base by using endovascular stents. J Neurosurg 95: 412-9, 2001
3. Halbach V et al: Aneurysms of the petrous portion of the internal carotid artery: Results of treatment with endovascular or surgical occlusion. AJNR 11: 253-7, 1990

Fibromuscular Dysplasia, Cervical

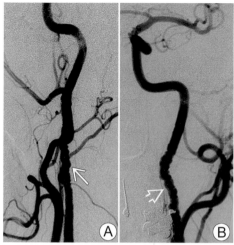

Fibromuscular dysplasia. (A) Lateral common carotid angio shows distal ICA long segment narrowing with characteristic "string-of-beads" appearance (arrow) of Type 1, FMD. (B) AP common carotid angio better delineates this cervical ICA area of FMD (open arrow). Notice typical sparing of intracranial ICA.

Key Facts
- Common acronym for fibromuscular dysplasia = **FMD**
- Definition: Arterial disease of unknown etiology affecting the medium & large arteries of young to middle-aged women
  - Arteriopathy = dysplastic arterial wall characterized by overgrowth of smooth muscle & fibrous tissue
- Classic imaging appearance
  - Angiography shows 3 distinct appearances
    - "String of beads" >> long tubular stenosis > asymmetric outpouching of one side of arterial wall
- Other key facts
  - Female predominance (90% in adults)
  - Most common arteries affected are renal arteries
  - Intracranial aneurysms present in 30% of patients with FMD
  - Spontaneous ICA dissection in ~ 20%
  - Vertebral artery involvement in 10%

Imaging Findings
<u>General Features</u>
- Best imaging clue
  - Multifocal, bilateral cervical ICA **"string of beads"** stenoses
- Lesions most common found at 1st & 2nd vertebral body level
<u>Digital Subtraction Angiography (DSA), CTA & MRA Findings</u>
- Most common: Multifocal stenosis, "ring-like" ridges, or "string of beads"
- Other appearances: Single, long, tubular stenosis & asymmetric outpouching of one side of arterial wall
- Complications that may be seen on angio, CTA or MRA
  - ICA occlusion (dissection); ICA pseudoaneurysm
- Angiographic classification
  - Type 1 (85%): Typical "string of beads"; medial fibroplasia

Fibromuscular Dysplasia, Cervical

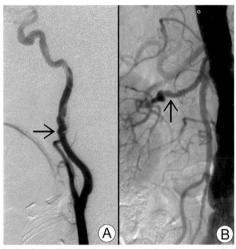

Fibromuscular dysplasia. (A) Lateral common carotid angiogram reveals characteristic "string-of-beads" appearance and irregularity of proximal internal carotid artery (arrow). (B) Renal angiogram shows similar typical findings of FMD of the right renal artery (arrow). (Courtesy Richard Wiggins MD)

- o Type 2 (~ 10%): Long tubular stenosis; intimal fibroplasia
- o Type 3 (~ 5%): Asymmetric outpouching along one side of ICA

Ultrasound Findings
- Distinguishing findings seen only in cases of excellent resolution
- Visible ridges or thickening of carotid wall, with or without stenosis
- Elevated velocity & disturbed flow in areas of stenosis
- Abnormal supra-bifurcation ICA in young women should make you suspect FMD

Imaging Recommendations
- DSA remains "gold standard" diagnostic modality
- MRA & CTA for noninvasive assessment, less accurate than DSA
- 3D contrast-enhanced MRA required for accurate diagnosis
- If FMD found in any artery, cervical & intracranial circulation should be studied for FMD & aneurysm respectively

Differential Diagnosis: Cervical ICA Stenosis

Atherosclerosis
- Older vasculopath
- Does not produce concentric ridges or "string of beads" appearance
- Usually focal, solitary stenosis at or above carotid bifurcation
- Type 3 FMD may mimic

ICA Dissection
- Posttraumatic or spontaneous
- Type 2 FMD may mimic

Takayasu Arteritis
- Large vessel arteritis

Fibromuscular Dysplasia, Cervical

Pathology

General

- General Path Comments
  - o **Dysplastic disorder**, not degenerative or inflammatory
  - o May affect other medium-size arteries (peripheral, abdominal, cephalic)
  - o Alternating zones of hyperplasia & weakening
    - Narrowing & dilatation = "sting-of-beads" appearance
  - o Weakened areas may cause aneurysm formation or dissection
- Genetics
  - o Not classical genetic disorder
  - o Familial in 11% of cases
- Epidemiology
  - o Renal artery >> internal carotid > others (lumbar, mesenteric, celiac, hepatic, iliac arteries)
  - o In US, FMD incidence is 0.6% from angio data & 1.1% from autopsy
  - o 4.4% asymptomatic incidence of FMD in adult renal transplant donors
- Etiology-Pathogenesis
  - o Unknown
  - o Alpha-1 antitrypsin deficiency, hormonal effects on smooth muscle & mural ischemia in dysplastic vessels = current hypotheses

Gross Pathologic

- Vessels shows alternating aneurysmal outpouching & stenoses

Histopathology

- Overgrowth of smooth muscle cells & fibrous tissue within arterial wall
- Three principal histopathologic varieties
  - o **Medial fibroplasia**: Medial layer involvement (85%)
  - o Periadventitial fibrosis: Involvement of adventitia adjacent to media
  - o Intimal fibroplasia: Intimal involvement

Clinical Issues

Presentation

- Most common presenting symptom: Transient ischemic attack
- Other presenting symptoms
  - o Renovascular hypertension (most common symptom overall)
  - o Stroke
- Demographics
  - o Age of onset: 25-50 years
  - o Gender predilection: Male to female ratio is 1:3
    - May present at any age, overlaps atherosclerosis age range

Treatment

- Antiplatelet ± anticoagulant therapy = conservative management
- Balloon angioplasty ± stenting is treatment of choice in patients with hemodynamically significant stenoses
- Surgical bypass used infrequently

Prognosis

- Guarded, slowly progressive disorder
- Long-term angioplasty results still pending

Selected References
1. Beregi JP et al: Fibromuscular dysplasia of the renal arteries: Comparison of helical CT angiography and arteriography. AJR 72: 27-34, 1999
2. Van Damme H et al: Fibromuscular dysplasia of the internal carotid artery: Personal experience with 13 cases and literature review. Acta Chir Belg 99: 163-8, 1999
3. Stewart MT et al: The natural history of carotid dysplasia. Vasc Surg 3: 305-10, 1986

Jugular Vein Thrombosis

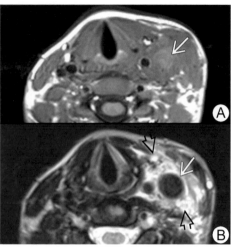

Jugular vein thrombophlebitis. (A) T1WI at level of cricoid reveals high-signal (methemoglobin) clot in thrombosed IJV (arrow). (B) T2WI shows clot to be low signal (arrow). Inflammatory edema surrounding vein is seen as high signal in adjacent soft tissues (open arrow). (Courtesy H Ric Harnsberger MD)

Key Facts
- Definitions
  - **Jugular vein thrombophlebitis (JVT)**: Acute to subacute thrombosis of internal jugular vein (IJV) with associated adjacent tissue inflammation (myositis and fasciitis)
  - **Jugular vein thrombosis**: Chronic IJV thrombosis (> 7 days) where clot persists within lumen but soft-tissue inflammation gone
- JVT presents to radiologists in its acute phase as "rule out abscess"; in its chronic phase, as "evaluate tumor extent"
- Classic imaging appearance: Luminal clot is present in most, or all, of IJV with soft-tissue inflammatory changes when acute-subacute

Imaging Findings
General Features
- Best imaging clue: Clot seen in IJV lumen
- Findings depend on the stage of the disease
- **Acute-subacute thrombophlebitic phases** (< 7 days): Imaging shows inflammation-induced loss of soft-tissue planes surrounding the enlarged, thrombus-filled IJV with vein wall rim enhancement
- **Chronic thrombotic phase** (> 7 days): Imaging shows a well-marginated, tubular mass without adjacent inflammation
  - Multiple venous collaterals are seen bypassing the thrombosis
- Edema fluid may be present in retropharyngeal space (RPS) as a secondary sign of JVT

CT Findings
- Acute-subacute thrombophlebitic phase: CECT shows increased density in fat surrounding carotid space (CS) secondary to cellulitis
  - IJV is enlarged and filled with low-density thrombus
  - Vasa vasorum of IJV wall enhances as a thin, hyperdense rim

Jugular Vein Thrombosis

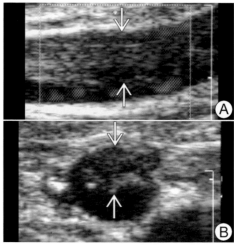

Jugular vein thrombosis. Long axis (A) and short axis (B) ultrasound images of subacute thrombus (arrows) in the internal jugular vein.

- Chronic thrombotic phase: Enhanced CT shows a tubular mass where the IJV should live without increased density in adjacent fat

MR Findings
- Acute-subacute phase: May have a bizarre tumorous appearance, especially on coronal plane; adjacent fat appears infiltrated
- Subacute to chronic phase: Tubular mass in the posterolateral CS with high signal on T1 images secondary to T1 shortening from the paramagnetic effect of methemoglobin
- MRV will show absent signal throughout most of the IJV

Ultrasound Findings
- Acute: Distended vein filled with hypoechoic thrombus
- Subacute/chronic: Decreased vein size, increased thrombus echogenicity, variable recanalization

Imaging Recommendations
- Ultrasound or CECT in these sick patients permits rapid diagnosis of JVT

Differential Diagnosis: Infrahyoid Neck CS Mass
Slow or Turbulent Flow in IJV
- High signal intensity on T1 MR images may be seen
- Look at all sequences, usually one will show flow
- If not, consider MRV to work this out

Reactive Adenopathy-Lymphadenitis
- Multiple focal masses along CS course of cervical neck

Cervical Neck Abscess
- Focal walled-off fluid collection in any space of infrahyoid neck

SCCa Malignant Adenopathy
- Multiple focal, necrotic, and non-necrotic masses along the course of the cervical CS and posterior cervical space

Jugular Vein Thrombosis

Pathology

General
- General Path Comments
  - JVT is different from intraparenchymal hematoma
  - In JVT there is lamination of thrombus, no hemosiderin deposition, and a delay in evolution of blood products (especially methemoglobin)
  - **Lemierre's syndrome**
    - Septic thrombophlebitis of IJV associated with disseminated metastatic abscesses in wake of an acute oropharyngeal infection in a young patient
    - Fusobacterium necrophorum, an obligate anaerobic, pleomorphic, gram-negative rod is grown from the blood or pus of these patients
- Pathogenesis: 3 mechanisms for thrombosis
  - Endothelial damage from an indwelling line or infection, altered blood flow and a hypercoagulable state
  - Venous stasis from compression of the IJV in the neck (nodes) or mediastinum (SVC syndrome) can also incite thrombosis
  - Migratory IJV thrombophlebitis (Trousseau syndrome) associated with malignancy (pancreas, lung and ovary)
    - Elevated factor VIII and accelerated generation of thromboplastin cause the hypercoagulable state

Clinical Issues

Presentation
- Principal presenting symptom: Swollen lateral infrahyoid neck
- Clinical diagnosis is unreliable
- Patient's history
  - Previous neck surgery, central venous catheterization, drug abuse, hypercoagulable state or malignancy
  - May be spontaneous clinical event
- **Acute thrombophlebitic phase**: Tender, red mass with low-grade fever; radiology requisition often reads "rule-out abscess"
- **Chronic thrombotic phase**: Hard, nontender mass; requisition reads "evaluate tumor extent"

Natural History
- IJV thrombophlebitis gives way to thrombosis over a 7-14 day period with decreased soft-tissue swelling

Treatment & Prognosis
- Aggressive antibiotics are given to treat any underlying infection; surgical drainage of focal pus is completed if seen on CT
- As clinically significant thromboembolism to the lungs is relatively rare in IJV thrombosis, anticoagulant therapy is usually not used
- Prognosis is related to the underlying cause of the IJV thrombosis
- IJV thrombosis itself is self-limited, with venous collaterals forming to circumvent the occluded vein

Selected References
1. Poe LB et al: Acute internal jugular vein thrombosis associated with pseudoabscess of the retropharyngeal space. AJNR 16: 892-6, 1995
2. Albertyn LE et al: Diagnosis of internal jugular vein thrombosis. Radiology 162: 505-8, 1987
3. Erdman WA et al: Venous thrombosis: clinical and experimental MR imaging. Radiology 161: 233-8, 1986

Juvenile Angiofibroma

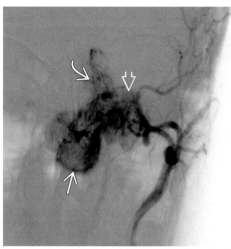

Juvenile angiofibroma. Left internal maxillary angiogram shows the intense tumor blush characteristic of juvenile angiofibroma, nasal (arrow), pterygopalatine fossa (open arrow) and sphenoid sinus (curved arrows) components of this tumor are identified.

Key Facts
- Synonyms: Juvenile nasopharyngeal angiofibroma (JNA); fibromatous or angiofibromatous hamartoma
  - JNA commonly used term but tumor begins in nose, (not in nasopharynx) and spreads secondarily into nasopharyngeal airway
  - Juvenile angiofibroma of the nasal cavity is a more correct terminology
- Definition: Vascular, non-encapsulated, benign nasal cavity mass that is found exclusively in **adolescent males**
- Classic imaging appearance: Heterogeneous, intensely enhancing nasal cavity, nasopharyngeal, maxillary and ethmoid sinus mass extending into pterygopalatine fossa, masticator space and orbit

Imaging Findings
General Features
- Best imaging clue: Posterior nasal mass in a young male
- Benign, vascular, locally aggressive nasal cavity mass
- Centered in posterior wall of nasal cavity, **at margin of sphenopalatine foramen**
- Penetrates the pterygopalatine fossa (PPF) early
- Early involvement of upper medial pterygoid lamina
CT Findings
- Bone remodeling ± destruction
- Ipsilateral nasal cavity and PPF enlarged
- Posterior wall maxillary sinus bowed anteriorly
- If large, penetration of vidian canal ± foramen rotundum conveys tumor into pterygoid plate and medial middle cranial fossa respectively
MR Findings
- Heterogeneous on both T1 and T2 MR images
- Multiple flow voids on T1 C- MR

Juvenile Angiofibroma

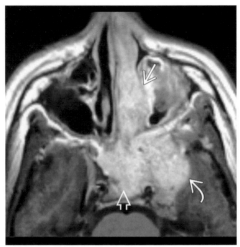

Juvenile angiofibroma. Axial T1 enhanced MR through the mid-maxillary sinus shows the avidly enhancing angiofibroma in the nose (arrow), sphenoid sinus (open arrow) and medial middle cranial fossa (curved arrow). This lesion is on the invasive end of the tumor spectrum.

- T1 C+ MR shows intense enhancement
- Coronal T1 C+ MR images necessary to show cavernous sinus, sphenoid sinus, or skull base extension

Plain Film Findings
- Lateral plain film of face shows anterior displacement of posterior wall of maxillary antrum associated with nasal opacification

Catheter Angiography
- Intense capillary blush is fed by enlarged feeding vessels from ECA
- **Internal maxillary**, ascending pharyngeal arteries from ECA are most common feeding vessels
  - o Supply may be from contralateral ECA branches as well
- If skull base/cavernous sinus extension, ICA supply is common

Imaging Recommendations
- Ideal workup to stage and characterize JAF includes
  - o Maxillofacial MR with T1 C+ in axial and coronal planes
  - o Bone-only non-contrasted CT in axial and coronal planes
  - o Catheter angiography of both ECA and ICA bilaterally
    - ▪ Helps plan surgery
    - ▪ Embolization of JAF decreases intra-operative blood loss

Differential Diagnosis: Mass in Nasal Cavity of Young Male
Nasal Polyp
- Does not have aggressive bone destruction
- Enhances only peripherally

Antrochoanal Polyp
- Maxillary antrum is full; PPF not involved
- Lesion herniates into anterior nasal cavity, then nasopharynx
- Peripheral enhancement only

Rhabdomyosarcoma
- Homogeneous mass with bone destruction

Juvenile Angiofibroma

- Not centered in posterolateral nasal cavity
- Does not usually penetrate the sphenopalatine foramen into PPF

Pathology

General

- General Path Comments
  - Angiomatous tissue in a fibrous stroma
- Etiology-Pathogenesis
  - Source of fibrovascular tissue of JAF is not known
  - Best current hypothesis: Primitive mesenchyme of sphenopalatine foramen is the source of JAF
- Epidemiology
  - 5-20% extend to skull base, and may have skull base erosion

Gross Pathologic or Surgical Features

- Reddish-purple, compressible, mucosa-covered, nodular mass
- Cut surface has a "spongy appearance"

Microscopic Features

- Vascular and fibrous tissue
  - **Myofibroblast** is cell of origin
  - Fibrovascular stroma, with fine neovascularity
  - May be purely fibrous, with reduced vascularity
- Estrogen, testosterone or progesterone receptors may be present

Clinical Issues

Presentation

- Principal presenting symptom: Unilateral nasal obstruction
- Other symptoms
  - Epistaxis
  - Pain or swelling in the cheek
- Adolescent male with average age at onset = 15 years
- 10-25 yrs reported age range

Natural History

- May rarely spontaneously regress

Treatment

- Complete surgical resection using pre-operative embolization to decrease blood loss
- Radiation therapy
  - Adjuvant to surgery
  - Recommended for intracranial extension, incomplete resection or local recurrence
- Hormonal therapy
  - Not routine, as complete tumor regression does not occur
  - Feminization side-effects undesirable in adolescent male

Prognosis

- Local recurrence rate with surgery 6-24%
- Local recurrence higher with large lesions, intracranial spread

Selected References
1. Gullane PJ et al: Juvenile angiofibroma: A review of the literature and a case series report. Laryngoscope 102: 928-33, 1992
2. Harrison DF: The natural history, pathogenesis, and treatment of juvenile angiofibroma. Arch Otolaryngol Head Neck Surg 113: 936-42, 1987
3. Lloyd GA et al: Juvenile angiofibroma: Imaging by magnetic resonance, CT and conventional techniques. Clin Otolaryngol 11: 247-59, 1986

Carotid Body Paraganglioma

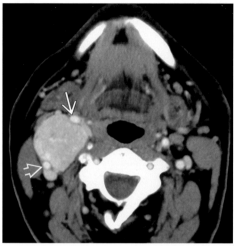

Carotid body paraganglioma. Axial contrast-enhanced CT shows the avidly enhancing tumor mass in the notch between the ECA (arrow) and the ICA (open arrow). The ECA and ICA are significantly splayed apart by this tumor. (Courtesy H Ric Harnsberger MD)

Key Facts
- Synonyms: Carotid body tumor, chemodectoma, non-chromaffin paraganglioma
- Definition: Carotid body paraganglioma (CBP) is a benign vascular tumor derived from primitive neural crest tissue located in the glomus bodies, in the crotch of the ECA and ICA at the carotid bifurcation
- Classic imaging appearance: Oropharyngeal carotid space mass splaying the ECA and ICA at the carotid bifurcation; avid enhancement with CT, high velocity flow voids on T1 MR, highly vascular on color Doppler US

Imaging Findings
General Features
- Best imaging clue: ECA and ICA are splayed
- Highly vascular mass is centered in the crotch of the carotid bifurcation
- ICA is characteristically displaced posterolaterally
- CT, MR and US appearances are diagnostic
CT & MR Findings
- Avidly-enhancing mass in the crotch between the ECA and ICA at the carotid bifurcation
- T1 MR images show "salt and pepper"
  - "Salt" is high-signal areas within the tumor parenchyma; secondary to subacute hemorrhage (seen only in larger tumors)
  - "Pepper" is punctate or curvilinear, low-signal foci from the high-velocity flow voids of feeding arteries (commonly seen)
- MRA will show splayed ECA-ICA but not the capillary bed of CBP
Ultrasound Findings (Color Doppler)
- Highly vascular tumor splaying the carotid bifurcation
- Possible invasion or stenosis of branch vessels
- Low resistance flow pattern in tumor vessels

Carotid Body Paraglioma

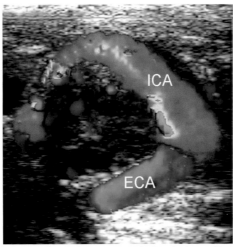

Carotid body paraganglioma. As seen on a color Doppler image, the internal- and external carotid arteries (ICA, ECA) are splayed by a typical, highly vascular paraganglioma.

Angiography Findings
- Enlarged feeding vessels with prolonged, intense vascular blush, with early draining veins seen secondary to arteriovenous shunting
- Ascending pharyngeal artery branches are principal tumor feeder

Imaging Recommendations
- In familial patient group, screening MR beginning at 20 years old
- MR and angiography done before surgery
- Angiographic challenges
  - To provide a vascular road map for the surgeon
  - Evaluate collateral arterial and venous circulation of the brain, should sacrifice of a major vessel become necessary
  - Search for multicentric tumors
  - Preoperative tumor embolization for prophylactic hemostasis

Differential Diagnosis: Cervical Carotid Space Mass

Carotid Bulb Ectasia
- Enlarged, ectatic, calcified carotid bulb secondary to atherosclerosis

Jugulodigastric (JD) Lymph Node Hyperplasia
- Enlarged, non-necrotic JD node pulsates against carotid bulb

Vagal Schwannoma
- MR shows fusiform enhancing mass in carotid space
- MRA shows ICA bowed over anterior surface of mass
- Absence of tumor blush or enlarged feeding arteries on angiography

Vagal Neurofibroma
- CECT shows low-density, well-circumscribed mass in carotid space (CS)
- MR imaging cannot differentiate from vagal schwannoma

Glomus Vagale Paraganglioma
- Mass centered approximately 2 cm below the skull base
- High-velocity flow voids on T1 MR images

Carotid Body Paraganglioma

Pathology
General
- Genetics
  - All paraganglioma occurs in a sporadic and a familial form
    - Familial paraganglioma is autosomal dominant
- Etiology-Pathogenesis
  - Arise from glomus bodies (paraganglia) in the carotid body
  - Glomus bodies are composed of chemoreceptor cells derived from the primitive neural crest
  - Glomus bodies are found in the temporal bone, jugular foramen and the upper carotid space to the level of the carotid bifurcation
- Epidemiology
  - CBP is the most common location for paraganglioma
  - 40% of all paragangliomas found are CBP
  - 5% of paragangliomas are multicentric in non-familial group
  - Familial incidence of multicentricity ~ 25%

Gross Pathologic or Surgical Features
- Lobulated, reddish-purple mass with fibrous pseudocapsule

Microscopic Features
- Chief cells and sustentacular cells are surrounded by a fibromuscular stroma
- Nests of chief cells are characteristic (zellballen)
- Electronmicroscopy shows neurosecretory granules

Clinical Issues
Presentation
- Principal presenting symptom: Pulsatile angle of mandible mass
- 20% have vagal and/or hypoglossal neuropathy
- Catecholamine-secreting CBP is rare

Treatment
- Surgical excision is treatment of choice
- Radiotherapy is used for lesion control in poor surgical candidates

Prognosis
- Untreated may destroy recurrent laryngeal nerve or invade carotid vessels with risk of stenosis or carotid rupture
- Low-grade malignant potential: 6% local recurrence, 2% distant metastasis
- Surgical cure without lasting post-operative cranial neuropathy is expected in CBP < 5 cm
- Complications of surgery, especially permanent vagal and/or hypoglossal neuropathy, increase with tumors > 5 cm

Selected References
1. Rao AB et al: Paragangliomas of the head and neck: Radiologic-pathologic correlation. RadioGraphics 19: 1605-32, 1999
2. Muhm M et al: Diagnostic and therapeutic approaches to carotid body tumors. Review of 24 patients. Arch Surg 132: 279-84, 1997
3. Olsen WL et al: MR imaging of paragangliomas. AJR 148: 201-4, 1987

Glomus Vagale Paraganglioma

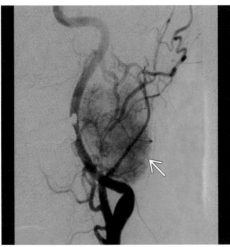

Glomus vagale paraganglioma. Common carotid angiogram viewed from laterally shows the highly vascular tumor (arrow) above the carotid bifurcation but below the skull base. The branches of the external carotid artery are enlarged and feed the tumor.

Key Facts
- Synonym: Vagal body tumors, glomus vagale
- Definition: Benign vascular tumor derived from primitive neural crest that begins in the ganglia of the vagus nerve
- Classic imaging appearance: **Nasopharyngeal carotid space mass** displacing the parapharyngeal fat anteriorly, the ICA anteromedial; avid enhancement with CT, high-velocity flow voids on T1 MR

Imaging Findings
General Features
- Mass is centered 1-2 cm below floor of jugular foramen in nasopharyngeal carotid space
- CS mass displaces parapharyngeal space anteriorly
- Internal carotid artery is displaced anteriorly or medially
- Both CT and MR are diagnostic

CT Findings
- Avidly-enhancing mass in nasopharyngeal CS

MR Findings
- **T1 MR** images show "salt and pepper"
- "Salt" or high-signal areas within the tumor parenchyma rarely seen; secondary to subacute hemorrhage
- "Pepper" is low-signal foci from the high-velocity flow voids of feeding arteries commonly seen; punctate or curvilinear

Angiography Findings
- Enlarged feeding vessels with prolonged, intense vascular blush with early draining veins seen secondary to arteriovenous shunting
- Ascending pharyngeal artery is principal tumor feeder

Imaging Recommendations
- In familial patient group, screening MR beginning at 20 years old
- MR and angiography done before surgery

Glomus Vagale Paraganglioma

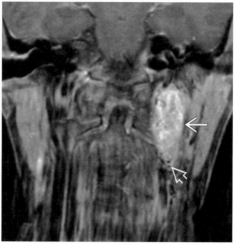

Glomus vagale paraganglioma. Coronal T1 enhanced, fat-saturated MR image reveals an ovoid avidly enhancing tumor (arrow) in the left carotid space. Notice that even with enhancement the high velocity flow voids (open arrow) can be seen along the tumor margin.

- Angiographic challenges
  - To provide a vascular road map for the surgeon
  - Evaluate collateral arterial and venous circulation of the brain, should sacrifice of a major vessel become necessary
  - Search for multicentric tumors
  - Preoperative embolization for prophylactic hemostasis

Differential Diagnosis: Nasopharyngeal Carotid Space Mass
<u>Vagal Schwannoma</u>
- MR shows fusiform enhancing mass in carotid space
- MRA shows ICA bowed over anterior surface of mass
- Absence of tumor blush or enlarged feeding arteries on angiography
<u>Meningioma of Carotid Space</u>
- Extends from jugular foramen above
- CT shows permeative sclerotic bony changes of the jugular foramen (JF) bony margins
- Dural thickening (tails) present along cephalad margin of JF
- Prolonged but mild tumor blush during angiography
<u>Glomus Jugular Paraganglioma</u>
- Mass centered in JF with permeative bony margins (CT) and high velocity flow voids (T1 MR)
<u>Carotid Body Paraganglioma</u>
- Mass centered in crotch of ICA-ECA at the carotid bifurcation
- T1 MR images show high-velocity flow voids

Pathology
<u>General</u>
- Genetics
  - Paraganglioma occurs in a sporadic and a familial form
    - The familial form is autosomal dominant

Glomus Vagale Paraganglioma

- Etiology-Pathogenesis
  - Arise from **glomus bodies = paraganglia**
  - Glomus bodies are composed of chemoreceptor cells derived from the primitive neural crest
- Epidemiology
  - Rarest of paragangliomas; 2.5% of all paragangliomas
  - 5% multicentric in non-familial group
  - Familial incidence of multicentricity may reach 90%

Gross Pathologic or Surgical Features
- Lobulated, reddish-purple mass with fibrous pseudocapsule

Microscopic Features
- Chief cells and sustentacular cells are surrounded by a fibromuscular stroma
- Nests of chief cells are characteristic (zellballen)
- Electronmicroscopy shows neurosecretory granules

Clinical Issues

Presentation
- Principal presenting symptom: Vocal cord paralysis
  - 50% have vocal cord paralysis at presentation
- Pulsatile lateral retropharyngeal mass
- Rarely hormonally active

Treatment
- Surgical excision is treatment of choice
- Radiotherapy is used for lesion control in poor surgical candidates
- If bilateral glomus vagale paraganglioma (GVP), surgery on one, radiotherapy on other to preserve unilateral vagus nerve function

Prognosis
- 100% have unilateral vagus nerve paralysis from surgery
- Teflon injection of ipsilateral vocal cord usually necessary
- Cricopharyngeal myotomy completed if dysphagia severe

Selected References
1. Rao AB et al: Paragangliomas of the head and neck: Radiologic-pathologic correlation. RadioGraphics 19: 1605-32, 1999
2. Urquhart AC et al: Glomus Vagale: Paraganglioma of the vagus nerve. Laryngoscope 104: 440-5, 1994
3. Olsen WL et al: MR imaging of paragangliomas. AJR 148: 201-4, 1987

Glomus Jugulotympanicum

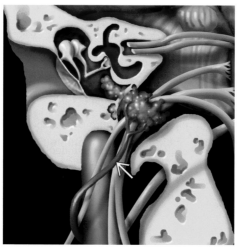

Glomus jugulotympanicum paraganglioma. Drawing shows the vascular mass of the superolateral jugular foramen invading into the middle ear cavity through the floor. The main arterial feeder is the ascending pharyngeal artery (arrow). The clinician sees only the tip of the iceberg behind the tympanic membrane.

Key Facts
- Synonyms: Glomus jugulare & jugulotympanicum paraganglioma
- Definition: **Glomus jugulotympanicum** describes paraganglioma involving both jugular foramen & middle ear cavity
- Classic imaging appearance
  - CT: **Permeative bone margins** of superolateral jugular foramen
  - MR: **High-velocity flow voids** on T1 NE MR
  - Angio: Rapid tumor blush & early venous egress
- Most common tumor found in jugular foramen

Imaging Findings
General Features
- Best imaging clue
  - Permeative-destructive walls of superolateral jugular foramen (JF) on CT of skull base
- **Glomus jugulotympanicum paraganglioma**
  - JF mass extends superolaterally into floor of middle ear cavity
  - Tumor spread **vector** is **superolateral** into middle ear cavity
CT Findings
- NECT: Permeative-destructive bone changes along superolateral margin of JF mark extent of tumor
  - Jugular spine erosion is common
  - Vertical segment of petrous ICA posterior wall often dehiscent
  - Mastoid segment of facial nerve may be engulfed
MR Findings
- **T1 NE MR** sequence show **"salt-and-pepper"** appearance
  - "Salt" or high-signal areas within the tumor parenchyma rarely seen
    - Secondary to subacute hemorrhage (methemoglobin)
  - "Pepper" = low-signal foci from high-velocity flow voids

Glomus Jugulotympanicum

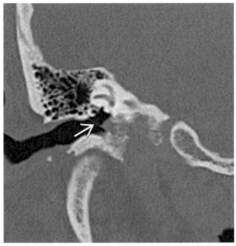

Glomus jugulotympanicum paraganglioma. Coronal CT of the right temporal bone shows the tumor spreading from the jugular foramen below superolaterally through the floor of the middle ear cavity. Permeative-destructive bone changes are characteristic. Tumor can be seen abutting the tympanic membrane (arrow).

- CE T1 MR
  - Will show true extent of tumor in skull base & middle ear cavity
  - May show tumor extending intraluminal with internal jugular vein
  - Coronal images show tongue of tumor curving up from JF, through middle ear floor, terminating on cochlear promontory

Angiography Findings
- Enlarged feeding vessels with **prolonged, intense, vascular blush** with early draining veins seen secondary to arteriovenous shunting
- Ascending pharyngeal artery = major feeding vessel

Imaging Recommendations
- CT, MR and angiography all done before surgery
- CT provides surgeon information about bony destruction, dehiscence, and landmarks not available from MR alone
- MR reveals exact soft tissue extent of tumor
- Angiography provides a vascular road map for surgeon
  - Evaluates collateral arterial & venous circulation of the brain
  - Searches for multicentric tumors
  - Embolization used for preoperative hemostasis

Differential Diagnosis: Jugular Foramen Mass
High-Riding Jugular Bulb
- JF bony margins intact
- Increased signal within bulb does not persist in all MR sequences
Dehiscent Jugular Bulb
- Sigmoid plate is focally dehiscent
- Polypoid extension into middle ear is contiguous with jugular bulb
Meningioma of JF
- NECT: Permeative-sclerotic bony changes
- CE T1 MR: Enhancing mass with dural tails
- Vector of spread: Centrifugal spread along dural surfaces

- Angio: Prolonged but mild tumor blush

Schwannoma of JF
- NECT: Smooth enlargement of JF
- CE T1 MR: Fusiform enhancing mass ± intramural cysts
- Vector of spread: Spreads along course of 9-11 cranial nerves
- Angio: Absence of tumor blush or enlarged feeding arteries on angiography; "puddling" on venous phase

Pathology

General
- Etiology-Pathogenesis
  - Arise from **glomus** (L. "a ball") **bodies = paraganglia**
    - Composed of chemoreceptor cells from primitive neural crest
- Epidemiology
  - Multicentric 5% of time
  - When familial, multicentricity reaches 25%

Gross Pathologic or Surgical Features
- Lobulated, solid mass with a fibrous pseudocapsule
- External surface is reddish-purple
- Cut surface shows multiple enlarged feeding arteries

Microscopic Features
- Biphasic cell pattern composed of **chief cells** & **sustentacular cells** surrounded by fibromuscular stroma
  - Chief cells arranged in characteristic compact cell nests or balls of cells (zellballen)
- Electronmicroscopy: Shows neurosecretory granules

Clinical Issues

Presentation
- Most common presenting symptom: Objective pulsatile tinnitus
- Other symptoms: 9-11 ± 12 cranial neuropathy; 7 or 8 cranial neuropathy less often
- Otoscopic exam: Vascular retrotympanic mass
- Demographics
  - Age: 40-60 years
  - Gender: Male:Female ratio = 3:1

Natural History
- Slow growing tumor can be watched in older patients

Treatment
- Surgery: Infratemporal fossa approach (Fisch Type A)
- Larger lesions may require surgery and radiation therapy
- Radiation therapy alone is palliative for older patients

Prognosis
- 60% of patients have postoperative cranial neuropathy

Selected References
1. Rao AB et al: Paragangliomas of the head and neck: Radiologic-pathologic correlation. RadioGraphics 19: 1605-32, 1999
2. Vogl TJ et al: Glomus tumors of the skull base: Combined use of MR angiography and spin-echo imaging. Radiology 192: 103-10, 1994
3. Olsen WL et al: MR imaging of paragangliomas. AJR 148: 201-4, 1987

Glomus Tympanicum

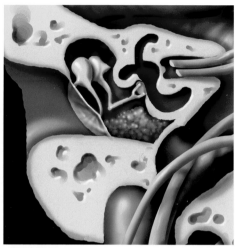

Drawing of GTP. The paraganglioma is depicted hanging from the lateral margin of the cochlear promontory. Its lateral margin abuts the tympanic membrane. No ossicle erosion is present. The floor of the middle ear cavity is intact.

Key Facts
- Synonym: Glomus tympanicum paraganglioma (GTP)
- Definition: Benign tumor that arises in glomus bodies situated on cochlear promontory of medial wall of middle ear cavity
- Classic imaging appearance: Round mass with base on cochlear promontory; CT shows no bone erosion and T1 C+ MR shows intense enhancement
- GTP may be clinically indistinguishable from glomus jugulotympanicum paraganglioma or AbICA; imaging must differentiate these diagnoses
- Most common tumor of middle ear cavity

Imaging Findings
General Imaging Features
- Best imaging clue: MR shows enhancing mass on cochlear promontory
- Floor of middle ear cavity is intact (if eroded, jugulotympanicum)

CT Findings
- Focal mass on cochlear promontory is characteristic
- Small lesions: Fills lower middle ear, just reaches medial border of tempanic membrane (TM)
- Large lesions: Fills middle ear cavity, creating attic block resulting in fluid collection in mastoid; margins of tumor not visible on CT
- Bone erosion **not** usually present with GTP, even with larger lesions
- Rare involvement of air cells along the inferior cochlear promontory may be mistaken for invasion

MR Findings
- T1 C+ MR shows focal enhancing mass on cochlear promontory
- Small GTP will be missed if slice thickness exceeds 3 mm
- Very large GTP may leave middle ear via eustachian tube

Angiography Findings
- Unnecessary if GTP diagnosis clearly established by CT

Glomus Tympanicum

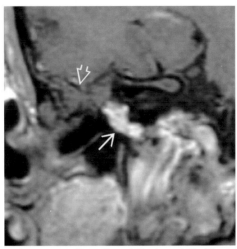

Glomus tympanicum paraganglioma. Coronal T1 enhanced MR of the right ear shows the avidly-enhancing glomus tympanicum tumor (arrow) filling the mesotympanum and hypotympanum. The floor of the middle ear cavity is not violated. Trapped fluid is lower in signal in the epitympanum (open arrow).

- GTP supplied by enlarged ascending pharyngeal artery and its inferior tympanic branch, via inferior tympanic canaliculus

Imaging Recommendations
- Bone-only CT without contrast best if GTP suspected clinically
- MR and angiography only used if glomus jugulotympanicum found by CT

Differential Diagnosis: Middle Ear Mass

Aberrant Internal Carotid Artery
- Imaging: Tubular mass crosses middle ear cavity to rejoin horizontal petrous ICA; large inferior tympanic canaliculus
- Clinical: Vascular mass behind TM ± pulsatile tinnitus

Dehiscent Jugular Bulb
- Imaging: CT shows sigmoid plate is dehiscent; venous protrusion into middle ear cavity from superolateral jugular bulb
- Clinical: Asymptomatic incidental otoscopic observation

Congenital Cholesteatoma of Middle Ear
- Imaging: C+ T1 MR shows no enhancement
- Clinical: "White" mass behind intact TM

Glomus Jugulotympanicum Paraganglioma
- Imaging: CT shows permeative change in bony floor of middle ear
- Clinical: Identical to GTP

Pathology

General
- Etiology-Pathogenesis
  - Arise from **glomus** (L. "a ball") **bodies** (paraganglia) found along inferior tympanic nerve (Jacobson's nerve) on cochlear promontory
    - Chemoreceptor cells derived from primitive neural crest
  - Nonchromaffin (nonsecretory) in this location
- Epidemiology

Glomus Tympanicum

- o GTP = most common tumor of middle ear
- o GTP **not** associated with multicentric paragangliomas

Gross Pathologic or Surgical Features
- Glistening, red polypoid mass with base on cochlear promontory
- Fibrous pseudocapsule

Microscopic Features
- Biphasic cell pattern composed of chief cells and sustentacular cells surrounded by fibromuscular stroma
- Chief cells arranged in characteristic compact cell nests or balls of cells
  - o Referred to as zellballen
- Immunohistochemistry: Chief cells show a diffuse reaction to chromogranin
- Electronmicroscopy: Shows neurosecretory granules

Glasscock-Jackson Classification of GTP
- Type I: Small mass limited to cochlear promontory
- Type II: Tumor completely filling middle ear space
- Type III: Tumor filling middle ear and extending into mastoid air cells
- Type IV: Tumor filling middle ear, extending into the mastoid or through tympanic membrane to fill the external auditory canal; may extend anterior to carotid artery

Clinical Issues

Presentation
- Principal presenting sign: Vascular retrotympanic mass
- Other symptoms: Pulsatile tinnitus (90%), conductive hearing loss (50%), facial nerve paralysis (5%) & asymptomatic (5%)
- Male: Female ratio = 1:3
- 66% are between 40-60 years of age at diagnosis
- Vascular (red) retrotympanic mass
  - o Anteroinferior quadrant of tympanic membrane

Natural History
- Slow-growing, non-invasive tumor
- Average time from onset of symptoms to surgical treatment is 3 years

Treatment
- Tympanotomy for smaller lesions; mastoidectomy for larger lesions
- Incomplete surgery of glomus jugulotympanicum paraganglioma or biopsy of an AbICA may result in serious patient complications
- The radiologist must correctly interpret the pretreatment images!

Prognosis
- Complete resection yields a permanent surgical cure

Selected References
1. Mafee MF et al: Glomus faciale, glomus jugulare, glomus tympanicum, glomus vagale, carotid body tumors, and simulating lesions: Role of MRI. Radiol Clin North Am 38: 1059-76, 2000
2. Larson TC et al: Glomus tympanicum chemodectomas: Radiographic and clinical characteristics. Radiology 163: 801-6, 1987
3. Lo WW et al: High-resolution CT in the evaluation of glomus tumors of the temporal bone. Radiology 150: 737-42, 1984

PocketRadiologist™
Vascular
Top 100 Diagnoses

SPINE

Spinal Cord Infarction

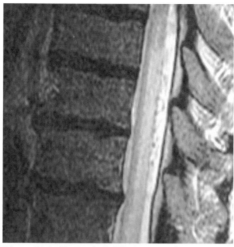

Sagittal T2WI in a patient with paraplegia following severe hypotension during surgery. Note diffuse cord swelling, hyperintensity.

Key Facts

- Definition: Permanent tissue loss in the spinal cord due to vascular occlusion, typically a radicular branch of the vertebral artery (cervical cord) or the aorta (thoracic cord and conus)
- Classic imaging appearance: T2 hyperintensity involving the anterior horn cells
- Other key facts
  - Most frequent in the upper thoracic cord because of arterial border zone
  - Sudden onset of neurologic deficits
  - Anterior spinal syndrome presents with paralysis, loss of pain and temperature sensation, and bladder and bowel dysfunction
  - Posterior spinal cord infarction characterized by loss of proprioception and vibration sense, paresis, and sphincter dysfunction
  - Anterior sulcus artery occlusion presents with Brown-Sequard syndrome

Imaging Findings

General Features

- Best imaging clue: Focal hyperintensity on T2WI in slightly expanded cord

MR Findings

- Normal or slightly enlarged spinal cord acutely
- Atrophy in late stage
- No significant T1 signal abnormality
- T2 hyperintensity in the gray matter, the gray matter with adjacent white matter, or the entire cross sectional area of the cord
- Focal hemorrhagic conversion may occur with hyperintensity on T1WI and hypointensity on T2WI
- Patchy post-gadolinium enhancement in subacute phase
- More sensitive than CT but not as specific due to CSF inflow effects in basal cisterns

Spinal Cord Infarction

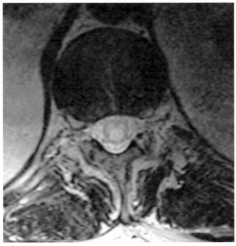

Same case as previous page. Axial T2WI shows the central gray matter, the cord watershed zone is markedly hyperintense.

- May see large vessel abnormalities such as aortic aneurysm or dissection
- Marrow T2 hyperintensity in the anterior vertebral body or in the deep medullary portion near the endplate may be present due to vertebral body infarct

Other Modality Findings
- Spinal artery occlusion on angiography
- Dissection or aneurysm in appropriate artery on MRA or catheter angiography

Differential Diagnosis

Multiple Sclerosis
- Dorsolateral in location
- Less than two vertebral segments in length
- Less than half the cross-sectional area of the cord
- 90% incidence of associated intracranial lesions on thin slice, sagittal FLAIR
- Relapsing and remitting clinical course

Spinal Cord Neoplasm
- Cord expansion invariably present
- Diffuse or nodular contrast enhancement
- Extensive peritumoral edema
- Associated cystic changes
- Slower clinical onset

Viral Myelitis
- Lesion centrally located
- 3 to 4 segments in length
- Occupying more than two thirds of the cord's cross-sectional area
- No associated intracranial lesions
- Onset not quite as sudden
- Clinically: "Transverse myelitis"

Spinal Cord Infarction

Pathology

General

- Embryology-Anatomy
  - Seven to eight of the 62 (31 pairs) radicular arteries supply the spinal cord in three territories
    - Cervicothoracic territory includes the cervical cord and the first two or three thoracic segments, supplied by anterior spinal artery from the vertebral artery and branches of the costocervical trunk
    - Midthoracic territory includes the fourth to eighth thoracic segments, supplied by a radicular branch from the aorta at the T7 level
    - Thoracolumbar territory includes the remainder of the thoracic segments and the lumbar cord, supplied by the artery of Adamkiewicz
  - The artery of Adamkiewicz usually originates from the 9th, 10th, 11th, or 12th intercostal artery (75%), less commonly from the higher intercostal artery or a lumbar artery
  - The radicular arteries form one anterior and two posterior spinal arteries
  - The anterior spinal arteries and branches supply the gray matter and an adjacent mantle of white matter
  - The posterior spinal arteries and branches supply one third to one half of the periphery of the cord
- Etiology-Pathogenesis
  - Idiopathic
  - Atherosclerosis
  - Thoracoabdominal aneurysm
  - Aortic surgery
  - Systemic hypotension
  - Infection
  - Embolic disease
  - Spinal arteriovenous malformation
- Epidemiology
  - Rare, usually patients > 50

Clinical Issues

Presentation

- Abrupt onset of weakness and loss of sensation
- Rapid progression of neurologic deficits, reaching maximum impairment within hours

Treatment

- Anticoagulation
- Intravenous corticosteroids
- Maintain systemic perfusion
- Physical rehabilitation

Prognosis

- Poor with limited recovery of neurologic function

Selected References
1. Yuh WT et al: MR imaging of spinal cord and vertebral body infarction. AJNR 13: 145-54, 1992
2. Berlit P et al: Spinal cord infarction: MRI and MEP findings in three cases. Journal of Spinal Disorders 5: 212-6, 1992
3. Mawad ME et al: Spinal cord ischemia after resection of thoracoabdominal aortic aneurysms: MR findings in 24 patients. AJNR 11: 987-91, 1990

Dural Arteriovenous Fistula, Spine

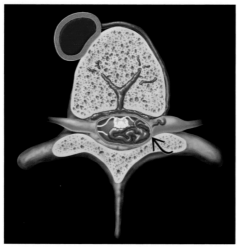

Intradural dorsal AVF, type A. Single arterial feeder enters the thecal sac through the left neural foramen root sleeve and drains through a dilated intradural vein via a single arteriovenous connection (arrow). Note conus compression, myelopathy.

Key Facts
- Synonym(s): DAVF, Dural AVF, Type I AVM
- Definition: Spinal AV fistula, usually dorsal intradural
- Classic imaging appearance: Abnormally enlarged and T2 hyperintense distal cord covered with dilated pial veins
- 80% of spinal vascular malformations
- Typical patient presents in third to sixth decade with progressive lower extremity weakness exacerbated by exercise
- No association with other CNS vascular malformations
- Imaging and clinical findings are frequently subtle or nonspecific; early diagnosis requires a high level of suspicion

Imaging Findings
General Features
- Most commonly occur at level of conus
- Best imaging clue: Small dilated pial veins on the dorsal or ventral surface of a swollen T2 hyperintense distal cord/conus
CT Findings
- Enlarged distal spinal cord
- Enhancing pial veins on cord surface
- Much more difficult to diagnose on CT than MR imaging
MR Findings
- T1WI: Cord enlargement and abnormal hypointensity
  - Abnormal small enhancing vessels on cord pial surface
- T2WI: Cord enlargement and abnormal hyperintensity
  - Multiple small abnormal vessel flow voids (dilated pial veins) on the cord pial surface
- Occasionally MR imaging is normal or demonstrates abnormal cord signal only

Dural Arteriovenous Fistula, Spine

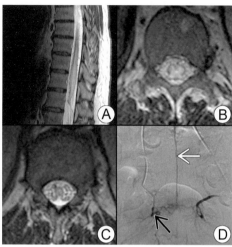

DAVF. Sagittal (A) and axial (B, C) T2WI show enlargement and abnormal T2 hyperintensity of the distal cord and conus representing venous hypertension. Note numerous pial vein flow voids. (D) Selective catheter angiogram reveals AVF (white arrow) with draining perimedullary vein (black arrow).

Other Modality Findings
- Spinal arteriography is gold standard for confirming diagnosis
  - Permits identification of exact level of arteriovenous shunt
  - Provides access for interventional therapy

Imaging Recommendations
- First perform focused MR imaging with small field of view and thin slices in both sagittal (3 mm/0 mm gap) and axial planes (4 mm/0 mm gap)
  - T1WI, T2WI, and enhanced T1WI sequences in both planes
- Use selective spinal arteriography to confirm diagnosis and direct treatment planning

Differential Diagnosis

Spinal Cord Arteriovenous Malformation (SCAVM)
- Usually acute presentation (compared to insidious presentation of DAVF)
- Intramedullary or subarachnoid hemorrhage relatively common

Amyotrophic Lateral Sclerosis
- Usually distinguished from DAVF by eliciting specific clinical features
- Brain MR imaging may be characteristically abnormal

Cervical or Thoracic Spondylosis/Disc Disease
- Distinguishable clinically and by imaging

Pathology

General
- General Path Comments
  - Lesions are extramedullary AVFs, not true AVMs
    - No intervening small vessel network
    - Fistula drains directly into venous outflow tract
    - Usually intradural
  - Supplied by small tortuous arteries originating from the dura mater

Dural Arteriovenous Fistula, Spine

- Etiology-Pathogenesis
  - o Postulated to be acquired lesions, possibly from thrombosis of extradural venous system
  - o Venous drainage from the DAVF results in increased pial vein pressure that is transmitted to the intrinsic cord veins
  - o Venous hypertension from engorgement reduces intramedullary AV pressure gradient, causing reduced tissue perfusion and cord ischemia
- Epidemiology
  - o 80% of patients are male
  - o Usually presents in 4th or 5th decade
    - Range: Ages 20s through 80s

Gross Pathologic or Surgical Features
- Most commonly occurs at the thoracolumbar level (T5-L3)
- Usually located either adjacent to the intervertebral foramen or within the dural root sleeve
- Arterial supply arises from dural branch of a radicular artery
- Intradural vein drains directly into the cord pial veins
- Frequently poor correlation between the location of the AV shunt and the clinical level of spinal dysfunction
- Rarely, clinically manifests as "subacute necrotizing myelopathy" ("Foux-Alajounine syndrome")

Staging or Grading Criteria
- Previously categorized as Type IV spinal arteriovenous malformation
  - o Misnomer that implies a true AVM etiology rather than AVF

Clinical Issues
Presentation
- Most common presentation is progressive lower extremity weakness with both upper and lower motor neuron involvement
- Additional symptoms include back pain, bowel/bladder dysfunction, and impotence
- Thoracolumbar fistula location spares upper extremities
- Never presents with hemorrhage

Natural History
- Slowly progressive clinical course over several years leading to paraplegia

Treatment
- Endovascular fistula occlusion with permanent embolic agents
- Surgical fistula obliteration

Prognosis
- Cord ischemia is reversible if treated early, but may become irreversible when untreated
- Bowel/bladder dysfunction and impotence rarely improve, even after successful obliteration of fistula

Selected References
1. Spetzler RF et al: Modified classification of spinal cord vascular lesions. J Neurosurg (Spine 2) 96: 145-56, 2002
2. Connors J et al: Interventional Neuroradiology. 1st ed. Philadelphia: W.B. Saunders, 1999
3. Anson J et al: Classification of spinal arteriovenous malformations and implications for treatment. BNI Quarterly 8: 2-8, 1992

Arteriovenous Malformation, Spine

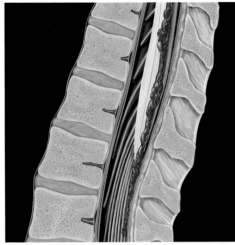

Sagittal graphic depicts a subpial juvenile (type III) cord AVM. Note "scalloped" appearance of the dorsal cord caused by enlarged draining veins. Chronic venous hypertension has caused cord atrophy.

Key Facts
- Definition: Direct arterial/venous communications without capillary bed
- Traditional classification
  - Type I: Dural arteriovenous fistula (DAVF)(See "Dural Arteriovenous Fistula, Spine")
  - Type II: Intramedullary glomus type AVM (similar to brain AVM)
  - Type III: Juvenile-type AVM (intramedullary, extramedullary)
  - Type IV: Intradural extra/perimedullary AVF (Types A, B, C)
- Newest classification of AVMs into extra-intradural; intradural (intramedullary, compact, diffuse, conus; subtyped by flow, size)
- AVMs account for < 10% of spinal masses
  - Most common = Type I (up to 80%)
  - Second most common = Intramedullary, Type II, III (15-20%)
- Imaging: Prominent "flow voids" + variable cord atrophy/gliosis

Imaging Findings
General Features
- Best imaging clue: Flow voids with cord hyperintensity (Type I)
  - Type II: Intramedullary nidus (may extend to dorsal subpial surface)
  - Type III: Nidus may have extramedullary and extraspinal extension
  - Type IV: Ventral fistula (venous varices displace, distort cord)
CT Findings
- NECT: Usually normal (rare = widened interpedicular distance, posterior vertebral scalloping)
- CECT: May show enlarged cord with enhancing nidus, pial vessels (rare)
MR Findings
- Types II, III (intramedullary AVMs)
  - T1WI: Large cord, heterogeneous signal (blood products), flow voids
  - T2WI: Cord hyperintense (edema, gliosis, ischemia) or mixed (blood)
  - Contrast enhanced T1WI: Variable enhancement of nidus, cord, vessels

Arteriovenous Malformation, Spine

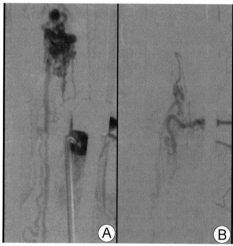

A 22-year-old female with scoliosis and progressive myelopathy after fixation. Spinal angiography demonstrates a compact vascular nidus supplied mostly by left T9 (A) radicular artery. Some supply comes from T8 (B). Type II (glomus) AVM.

- Type IV (perimedullary)
  - T1WI: Ventral fistula, large flow voids distort/displace cord
  - T2WI: Hyperintense cord + flow voids
  - Contrast: Enhancing pial vessels, epidural plexus, +/- patchy enhancement distal cord

Other Modality Findings
- DSA
  - Type II: Supplied by anterior spinal artery (ASA) or posterior spinal artery (PSA); nidus drains to coronal venous plexus (on cord surface) which in turn drains anterograde to extradural space
  - Type III: Large complex nidus, multiple feeding vessels; may be intramedullary and extramedullary and even extraspinal
  - Type IV: Feeding vessel from ASA or PSA connects directly with spinal vein (no nidus!)
- Myelography (intramedullary/perimedullary AVMs): Serpentine filling defects along posterior cord

Imaging Recommendations
- Contrast-enhanced MRI; consider spinal angiography +/- embolization

Differential Diagnosis
Intramedullary Neoplasm
- Ependymoma: Heterogeneous (cysts, blood products)
- Astrocytoma: Multisegmental enhancing mass, no enlarged vessels

Pathology
General
- General Path Comments
  - Location
    - Type II (glomus): Cervical/upper thoracic (may occur anywhere)
    - Type III (juvenile): Cervical/upper thoracic (may occur anywhere)

Arteriovenous Malformation, Spine

- Type IV: Conus medullaris (type A, B), thoracic (type C)
- Genetics (can be sporadic or syndromic)
  - Type II: Associated with cutaneous angiomas, Klippel-Trenaunay-Weber, Rendu-Osler-Weber syndromes
  - Type III: Associated with Cobb's syndrome (metameric vascular malformation involving triad of spinal cord, skin, bone)
  - Type IV: Associated with Rendu-Osler-Weber syndrome
- Embryology
  - Persistence of primitive direct communications between arterial and venous channels, without intervening capillary bed
- Etiology-Pathogenesis
  - Type II: Compact nidus, high-flow, aneurysms common (20-44%)
  - Type III: Large diffuse nidus, cord ischemia, venous hypertension
  - Type IV: Congenital; may be acquired after trauma; (A) venous hypertension, (B, C) arterial steal, (C) cord compression
- Epidemiology
  - Intramedullary (Type II, III): 15-20% of spinal AVM; Type IV: 10-20%

Gross Pathologic-Surgical Features

- Type II: Compact intramedullary nidus lacks normal capillary bed; no parenchyma within nidus; (nidus may have pial extension)
- Type III: Large, complex intramedullary lesion, normal neural parenchyma inside nidus (may involve extramedullary, extradural)
- Type IV: Direct fistula between ASA/PSA & draining vein, no nidus
  - IV-A: Small AVF with slow flow, mild venous enlargement
  - IV-B: Intermediate AVF, dilated feeding arteries; high flow rate
  - IV-C: Large AVF, dilated feeding arteries; dilated, tortuous veins

Microscopic Features

- Abnormal vessels with variable wall thickness, internal elastic lamina
- Reactive change in surrounding tissue: Gliosis, cytoid bodies, Rosenthal fibers; hemosiderin deposition common; +/- Ca++

Clinical Issues

Presentation

- Type II: M=F, 20-40y, SAH most common symptom; pain, myelopathy
- Type III: M=F, < 30y, progressive neurologic decline (weakness), SAH
- Type IV: M=F, 10-40y, progressive conus /cauda equina syndrome, SAH

Treatment

- Type II: Surgical resection, + pre-op embolization (aneurysms, nidus)
- Type III: Complete resection generally not possible, palliative therapy
- Type IV: Embolization or surgical resection: (A) surgical resection, (B) surgical resection or embolization, (C) embolization

Prognosis

- Good outcome in Type II (glomus) and IV (perimedullary)
- Poor prognosis for juvenile (Type III) AVM

Selected References
1. Spetzler RF et al: Modified classification of spinal cord vascular lesions. J Neurosurg (Spine 2) 96: 145-56, 2002
2. Bemporad JA et al: Magnetic resonance imaging of spinal cord vascular malformations with an emphasis on the cervical spine. In Neuropathic basis for imaging. Neuroimaging Clinics of North America 11: 111-29, 2001
3. Bao YH et al: Classification and therapeutic modalities of spinal vascular malformations in 80 patients. Neurosurgery 40: 75-81, 1997

PocketRadiologist™
Vascular
Top 100 Diagnoses

THORAX

Double Aortic Arch

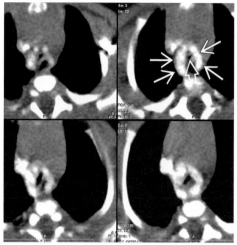

Double aortic arch shown in 3-day-old boy with stridor. Four consecutive axial, contrast enhanced CT section show persistent left and right (arrows) surrounding and severely compressing the trachea (open arrow). The right arch is larger than the left.

Key Facts
- Definition: Congenital arch anomaly related to persistence of both the left and right fourth aortic arches
- Classic imaging appearance: Severe compression of trachea with evidence of right and left arches
- Most common symptomatic vascular ring
- Airway compression usually severe
- Presentation typically early in life
- Typically an isolated lesion without associated anomalies

Imaging Findings
General Features
- Imaging evaluation includes radiography followed by cross-sectional imaging: CT or MRI
- Cross-sectional imaging performed to confirm diagnosis and define anatomic variations for pre-surgical planning
- Compression of the trachea, typically severe, at the level of the mid-trachea
- Esophagus also compressed
- On cross-sectional imaging, both left and right arches are identified arising from ascending aorta and joining to form descending aorta
- Each arch gives rise to a carotid and subclavian artery
- Right arch more commonly larger and more superior extending than left
- Esophogram no longer part of imaging workup
CT Findings
- Arches seen compressing trachea
- 3D images can be used to demonstrate arteriogram
MR Findings
- Axial images typically most helpful plane
- Arches seen compressing trachea

Double Aortic Arch

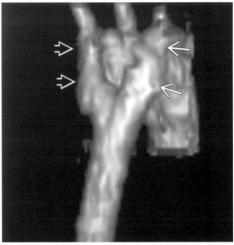

Double aortic arch shown in the same 3-day-old boy. 3D surface rendered CT arteriogram shows right (open arrows) and left (arrows) aortic arches arising from the ascending aorta and joining to form the descending aorta.

Radiography Findings
- Frontal radiographs show prominent soft tissue on either side of the trachea

Differential Diagnosis: Persistent Wheezing
Right Arch with Aberrant Left Subclavian Artery: Other Arch Abnormalities
- May not be possible to differentiate without cross sectional imaging
Aberrant Origin of the Left Pulmonary Artery
- Compression from posterior aspect of trachea on radiography
Nonvascular Masses
- Small middle mediastinal masses or larger anterior or posterior masses

Pathology
General
- Related to embryological persistence of the right and left 4th aortic arches
- True complete ring with trachea and esophagus engulfed

Clinical Issues
Presentation
- Patients typically present early in life, often soon after birth
- Severe stridor
- Most common symptomatic vascular ring
- Typically not associated with other congenital abnormalities (isolated lesion)
Treatment & Prognosis
- Thoracotomy with ligation of smaller of two arches
- Determination of which arch is smaller on cross-sectional imaging will determine which side thoracotomy is performed

- Up to 30% of patients may have persistent airway symptoms following initial surgical relief related to tracheomalacia, persistent extrinsic airway compression, or some combination of the two
- Some of these patients who have persistent symptoms may benefit from a second operation, such as aortopexy, other vascular suspension procedures, or airway resection or reconstruction
- 11% of patients required a second operation to relieve airway symptoms

Selected References
1. Donnelly LF et al: The spectrum of extrinsic lower airway compression in children: MR imaging. AJR 168: 59-62, 1997
2. Katz M et al: Spiral CT and 3D image reconstruction of vascular rings and associated tracheobronchial anomalies. J Comput Assist Tomogr 19: 564-8, 1995
3. Han MT et al: Double aortic arch causing tracheoesophageal compression. Am J Surg 165: 628-31, 1993

Innominate Artery Compression

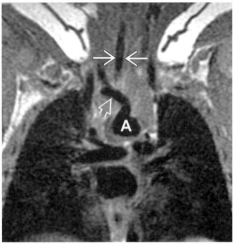

Innominate artery compression of the trachea in a 5-month-old-female. Coronal T1-weighted image shows the innominate artery (open arrow) arising to the left of the trachea (arrows) from the aortic arch (A). As the innominate artery crosses rightward, it compresses the trachea from anteriorly (see image on next page).

Key Facts
- Definition: The innominate artery passes immediately anterior to the anterior aspect of the trachea and leads to tracheal compression
- Classic imaging appearance: Narrowing of trachea from anterior compression just below thoracic inlet – best seen on lateral radiograph
- Controversial topic
- Spectrum of severity from severe compromise of trachea to minimal indentation on trachea (normal variation)
- Presentation includes stridor, apnea, dyspnea
- Disease of infants
- Symptoms will typically resolve as the child grows
- Surgery reserved for those with severe symptoms and who fail conservative management
- In infants, the innominate artery arises from the aortic arch to the left of the trachea
- In theory, this can in combination with the "crowded" anterior mediastinum (thymus) in infants lead to compression of the trachea as the innominate artery crosses obliquely rightward and ascends into the neck

Imaging Findings
CT and MR Findings
- Marked narrowing of the trachea in the superior mediastinum
- Tracheal narrowing confined to level at which the innominate artery crosses anterior to trachea
- Innominate artery immediately abuts area of tracheal narrowing
Radiography Findings
- On lateral radiography, compression from the anterior aspect of the trachea is present
- Compression is at level of superior trachea just below thoracic inlet

Innominate Artery Compression

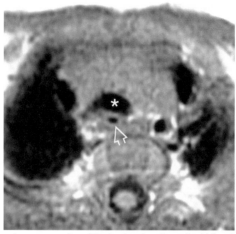

Innominate artery compression of the trachea in a 5-month-old female. Axial T1-weighted image shows the innominate artery (*) passing rightward anterior to the trachea. The trachea (arrow) is compressed at this level. The soft tissue anterior to the innominate artery is normal thymus.

- Left sided aortic arch identified
- Lung aeration not affected

Differential Diagnosis
<u>Duplication Cyst Compressing Airway</u>
<u>Lymphatic Malformation Compressing Airway</u>

Pathology
<u>General</u>
- In infants, the innominate artery arises from the aortic arch more to the left than it does in adults
- Superior mediastinum "crowded" in infants secondary to thymus
- Combination of these factors in theory leads to innominate artery compressing trachea as it passes rightward and anterior to trachea

Clinical Issues
<u>Presentation</u>
- Presentation is during infancy
- Presents with stridor, apnea, dyspnea
- Endoscopy shows fixed, pulsatile compression from the anterior aspect of the trachea just below thoracic inlet
<u>Natural History</u>
- The compression and resultant symptoms decrease over time as the child grows
<u>Treatment & Prognosis</u>
- Surgical therapy is controversial and reserved for those with severe symptoms and who fail conservative management
- Surgical aortopexy and re-implantation of innominate artery origin more rightward from the aortic arch

Innominate Artery Compression

- Persistent symptoms may be present after surgery if large component of tracheomalacia present

Selected References

1. Strife JL et al: Tracheal compression by the innominate artery in infancy and childhood. Radiology 139: 73-5, 1981
2. Berdon WE et al: Vascular anomalies and the infant lung: rings, slings, and other things. Semin Roentgenol 7: 39-63, 1972
3. Berdon WE et al: Innominate artery compression of the trachea in infants with stridor and apnea. Radiology 92: 272-8, 1969

Midline Descending Aorta

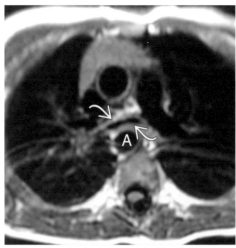

Midline descending aorta with airway compression in a 1-year-old boy. Axial T1-weighted MRI shows the descending aorta (A) to be in midline position, anterior to the vertebral bodies, rather than in a left paraspinal position. The tracheal carina (arrows) is compressed.

Key Facts
- Synonyms: Midline descending aorta – airway compression syndrome
- Definition
  - Descending aorta positioned immediately anterior to vertebral bodies rather than in normal left paravertebral location
  - Malposition leads to abnormal stacking of structures in the confined space between the spine and the anterior chest wall
- Classic imaging appearance: On cross-sectional imaging, aorta positioned immediately anterior to spine with associated airway compression
- The distal airway, most typically the carina or left main bronchus, is extrinsically compressed between the abnormally positioned descending aorta posteriorly and the pulmonary arteries anteriorly
- Occurs in infants and small children
- Can occur as an isolated lesion secondary phenomena associated with hypoplastic right lung and resultant mediastinal shift, right arch and left-sided descending aorta, double aortic arch, right aortic arch with left subclavian artery

Imaging Findings
MR and CT Findings
- Best demonstrated on axial CT or MRI images
- Descending aorta identified in position anterior to spine, rather than in paravertebral location
- Distal airway – typically carina or left main bronchus – compressed between malpositioned descending aorta posteriorly and pulmonary arteries anteriorly
- May be seen as isolated lesion

Midline Descending Aorta

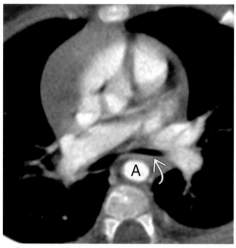

Midline descending aorta with airway compression in an 11-month-old boy. Contrast enhanced CT shows midline position of the descending aorta (A) anterior to the vertebral bodies, rather than in normal left paraspinal location. The left main bronchus (arrow) is compressed as a result.

- May be seen in association with hypoplastic right lung and resultant mediastinal shift, right arch and left sided descending aorta, double aortic arch, right aortic arch with left subclavian artery

Radiography Findings

- Radiographs often normal
- Radiographs insensitive to compression of the carina and proximal bronchi in children

Differential Diagnosis

Non-vascular Mediastinal Mass

- Small middle mediastinal masses such as duplication cyst, adenopathy

Other Atypical Vascular Causes of Compression

Pathology

General

- Etiology of isolated position of midline descending aorta unknown
- Descending aorta positioned immediately anterior to vertebral bodies rather than in normal left paravertebral location
- Malposition position leads to abnormal stacking of structures in the confined space between the spine and the anterior chest wall
- The distal airway, most typically the carina or left main bronchus, is extrinsically compressed between the abnormally positioned descending aorta posteriorly and the pulmonary arteries anteriorly

Clinical Issues

Presentation

- Typically present in infants
- Stridor
- Recurrent left-sided pneumonia

- Wheezing refractory to medical therapy
- Bronchoscopy demonstrates pulsatile, fixed compression of distal airway from posterior aspect
- Patients who have persistent respiratory symptoms after surgical therapy for double aortic arch may have airway compression secondary to midline descending aorta

Natural History
- Surgery reserved for severe cases
- Children will often grow out of compression over time

Treatment & Prognosis
- In severe cases, aortopexy may relieve symptoms by causing a re-shifting of the abnormally stacked anatomic structures

Selected References
1. Hungate RG et al: Left mainstem bronchial narrowing: A vascular compression syndrome? Evaluation by magnetic resonance imaging. Pediatr Radiol Jul 28: 527-32, 1998
2. Donnelly LF et al: The Spectrum of Extrinsic Lower Airway Compression In Children: MR Imaging. AJR 168: 59-62, 1997
3. Donnelly LF et al: Anomalous midline location of the descending aorta: a cause of compression of the carina and left mainstem bronchus in infants. AJR 164: 705-7, 1995

Takayasu's Arteritis

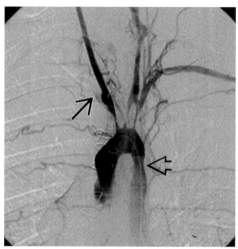

Extremely abnormal aorta and great vessels. The origins of all of the great vessels are stenotic. There is stenosis of the descending aorta (open arrow). The right subclavian artery is occluded (arrow).

Key Facts
- Synonym: Pulseless disease
- Definition: An idiopathic, systemic, granulomatous vasculitis which involves the aorta and its major branches
- Classic imaging appearance: Stenoses of large and medium sized arteries
- Multiple arteries involved: Great vessels, carotids, subclavian, pulmonary, renal, mesenteric, and coronary arteries, less commonly lower extremity
- Aneurysms may also occur in the affected arteries

Imaging Findings
General Features
- Best imaging clue: Stenoses of multiple arteries, relatively smooth narrowing
- Other radiographic features
  - Stenosis and occlusion of aorta (may mimic coarctation)
  - Thickening of aortic and arterial walls
  - Pulmonary artery involvement (50%), very specific if present
- Active disease: Early and delayed mural enhancement
- Inactive disease: Lack of mural enhancement, high attenuation pre-contrast, wall calcifications
CT Findings
- Aneurysms, mural changes, infiltration of adjacent mediastinal fat, loss of sharp vessel definition, aortic wall calcification
- Without contrast: Higher attenuation thickened arterial walls
- With contrast: "Double ring" pattern of aortic wall thickening
MR Findings
- Possible MR protocol: T2-weighted, pre- and post-intravenous contrast T1-weighted spin echo, MRA 2D time-of-flight, and 3D angiography with contrast

Takayasu's Arteritis

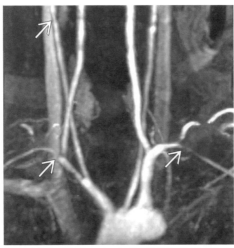

Gadolinium enhanced MRA of Takayasu's arteritis. Multiple stenoses in upper extremity arteries (arrows). Gadolinium markedly improves the signal-to-noise ratio and thus the image quality. (Courtesy John Kaufman MD)

- Aneurysms, mural changes, infiltration of adjacent mediastinal fat, loss of sharp vessel definition, aortic wall enhancement with contrast
- Misses subtle calcifications

Ultrasound Findings
- Demonstrates mural and luminal changes
- Assess hemodynamic effects of disease

Angiography Findings
- Stenoses and aneurysmal changes in multiple arteries
- If disease not active, normal ESR, angioplasty and/or stenting is option

Imaging Recommendations
- MRI/MRA - multiple imaging planes is ideal
- CT detects aneurysms, assess wall thickness
- Comprehensive angiogram evaluates disease extent, guides percutaneous or surgical therapy

Differential Diagnosis
Giant Cell Arteritis
- Older patient population
- Predilection for extracranial branches of the carotid artery

Pathology
General
- General Path Comments
  - Vessel findings range from acute inflammatory phase to old scarring
  - Degree of aortic involvement variable
  - Aortic root dilation may cause aortic valve insufficiency
- Etiology-Pathogenesis
  - Unknown etiology
  - Possibly infectious (links to tuberculosis)
  - Rheumatic etiology due to increased ASO, clinical signs/symptoms

Takayasu's Arteritis

- o Immune-mediated etiology proposed
- Epidemiology
  - o Predominant sex: Female > Male (9:1)
  - o Predominant age: < 30 years (90%)

Gross Pathologic or Surgical Features
- Marked aortic thickening and wall rigidity due to 3-layer fibrosis
- Stenosis or lumen narrowing
- Skip lesions
- Longitudinal wrinkling and ridging – "tree bark" appearance

Microscopic Features
- Acute phase
  - o Prominent granulomatous arteritis with giant cells
  - o Principally restricted to media and adventitia
- Inflammatory reaction
  - o Collagenous fibrosis involving all layers
  - o Lymphocytic infiltration

Staging or Grading Criteria
- Several grading methodologies
  - o Type I: Classic pulseless disease, Type II: Mixed type, Type III: Atypical coarctation, Type IV: Dilated type
  - o Type 1: Aortic arch, Type 2: Abdominal aorta, Type 3: Entire aorta, Type 4: Pulmonary arteries

Clinical Issues

Presentation
- Features of vascular occlusion
  - o Absent, decreased, or unequal pulses in limbs or carotid vessels, vascular bruits, claudication in limbs
  - o Hypertension, mesenteric ischemia or infarction
  - o Visual disturbances/retinopathy, syncope, stroke
  - o Angina, pulmonary hypertension, heart failure

Natural History
- Acute inflammation (non-specific features of inflammation)
- Fever, weight loss, tachycardia
- Vascular occlusion after having disease for 6-10 years

Treatment & Prognosis
- Medical treatment
  - o Active phase: Glucocorticoids
  - o Occlusive phase: Treat hypertension (HTN) and other complications
  - o Cyclophosphamide, methotrexate when glucocorticoids refractory or contraindicated
- Angioplasty and/or stenting for stenosis of aorta/large branches
- Surgery for significance symptomatic lesions
- Course is progressive over months or years for most individuals
- Overall survival at 10 years is 80%
- Severe HTN is a poor prognostic factor

Selected References
1. Atalay MK et al: Magnetic resonance imaging of large vessel vasculitis. Curr Opin Rheumatol 13:41-7, 2001
2. Sharma BK et al: Follow-up study of balloon angioplasty and denovo stenting in Takayasu arteritis. Int J Cardiol 75:S147-52, 2000
3. Matsunaga H et al: Takayasu arteritis: Protean radiologic manifestations and diagnosis. Radiographics 17: 579-94, 1997

Marfan Syndrome (MFS)

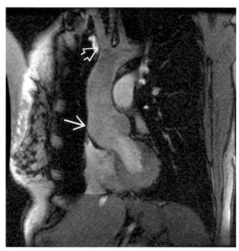

MRI of aortic root that demonstrates the typical dilatation of aortic sinuses of Valsalva. The appearance is referred to as "tulip bulb aorta" (arrow). Continued dilatation leads to aortic regurgitation. Incidentally noted is bovine arch configuration with conjoined innominate & left common carotid (open arrow).

Key Facts
- Definition: Multiorgan heritable connective tissue disorder characterized by cystic medial necrosis of large, medium-sized arteries
- Classic imaging appearance
  - Dilatation of aortic root and sinotubular junction causing "tulip bulb aorta" or "pear shaped" aorta
  - +/- Fusiform arteriopathy, saccular aneurysms
- Acute dissection: Very high mortality, necessitates emergency surgery
- Use transesophageal echocardiography (TEE) for rapid, safe assessment

Imaging Findings
General Features
- Best imaging clue: Dilated ascending aorta in patient with lens dislocation or "Marfanoid" skeletal features
CT Findings
- NECT
  - Aneurysmal dilatation of aortic root
  - +/- Enlarged great vessels
  - Intramural hematoma (with dissection)
- CECT: Strong, uniform enhancement; look for membrane separating true from false lumen
MR Findings
- T1WI: Variable depending on flow, age of intramural hematoma
- T2WI: Variable
- Other sequences
  - MR flow mapping may show decreased aortic distensibility, increased flow wave velocity
  - Spine MR may show dural ectasia, meningoceles
Other Modality Findings
- Angiography (DSA, MRA, CTA)

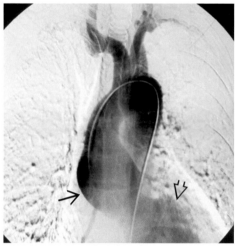

Typical dilatation of aortic sinuses of Valsalva. The appearance is referred to as "tulip bulb aorta" (arrow). As the aortic sinuses dilate aortic regurgitation develops (open arrow). The innominate artery is also dilated. (Courtesy Tom Kinney MD)

- o Annuloaortic ectasia: Involves sinus of Valsalva, ascending aorta
- o +/- Dissection
- o Less common
  - ▪ Fusiform dilatation of great vessels
  - ▪ Cephalocervical dissection(s) +/- pseudoaneurysms
  - ▪ Intracranial aneurysm
- o Rare: Aortic rupture
- TEE
  - o Common: Increased diameter of aortic root
  - o Look for signs of dissection
    - ▪ Membrane present, separates true from false lumen
    - ▪ Rupture sites with to-and-fro flow
  - o Associated abnormalities
    - ▪ Aortic regurgitation
    - ▪ Pericardial effusion

Imaging Recommendations
- TEE; CTA or MRA

Differential Diagnosis

Ehlers-Danlos Syndrome Type IV (EDS-IV)
- No Marfanoid features
- Easy bruising, thin skin, characteristic facial features
- Intracranial aneurysms more common

Hyperhomocystinemia
- Many overlapping clinical features with MFS
- Mental deficiency, thromboemboli, **downward** lens dislocation
- Associated with nontraumatic spontaneous cervical artery dissection

Autosomal Dominant Polycystic Kidney Disease
- May present with spontaneous arterial dissections, intracranial aneurysms

- Visceral cysts

Pathology
General
- Fusiform enlargement of large (aorta), medium-sized arteries (great vessels); +/- dissection
- Genetics
  - Autosomal dominant inheritance
    - **FBN1** = gene for Marfan syndrome
    - Large size (65 codons); heterogeneous mutations
- Etiology-Pathogenesis
  - MFS is a type 1 fibrillinopathy
  - Fibrillin-1 mutation results in abnormal "building block" of microfibrils that are major component of vessel walls
  - Arterial walls are weakened, progressively enlarge, are prone to dissection, rupture
- Epidemiology: 1 in 5000
Gross Pathologic or Surgical Features
- Dilated aortic arch +/- dissection, rupture
- Spinal dural ectasia (may be striking)
Microscopic Features
- Cystic medial necrosis (CMN) = most common arterial lesion

Clinical Issues
Presentation
- Clinical diagnosis of Marfan syndrome
  - Cardiovascular manifestations
    - Dilatation of aortic root at sinus of Valsalva
    - Ascending aortic dissection +/- aortic valve regurgitation
    - Floppy valve syndrome (mitral prolapse)
  - Ocular: **Upward** lens dislocation, myopia
  - Skeletal
    - Tall stature, span > height, pectus carinatum/excavatum, long slender limbs with arachnodactyly
    - Dilated spinal dura +/- radicular cysts, meningoceles
Natural History
- Common: Aneurysmal dilatation of aortic root
  - Begins in first or second decade
  - Premature death from aortic rupture, dissection, or cardiac complications of aortic regurgitation
- Less common: Spontaneous cephalocervical dissections, pseudoaneurysms form
Treatment & Prognosis
- Beta-adrenergic receptor inhibitors
- Emergent surgical repair if dissection, rupture
- Death due to aortic dissection, rupture

Selected References
1. Ho NC et al: Dural ectasia associated with Marfan syndrome. Radiol 223: 767-71, 2002
2. Groenink M et al: Biophysical properties of the normal-sized aorta in patients with Marfan syndrome: Evaluation with MR flow mapping. Radiol 219: 535-40, 2001
3. Schievink WI et al: Intracranial aneurysms in Marfan's syndrome: An autopsy study. Neurosurg 41: 866-71, 1997

Mycotic Aneurysm

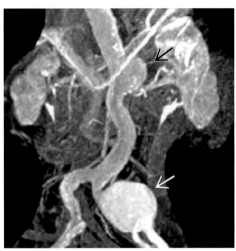

Mycotic aneurysm. 3D contrast MRA demonstrates multiple saccular aneurysms involving the aorta and left common iliac artery (arrows). This patient presented with flank pain and low-grade fever.

Key Facts
- Synonym: Infectious aneurysm (more appropriate term)
- Definition: Aneurysm arising from infection of arterial wall, usually bacterial
- Classic imaging appearance: Saccular aneurysm arising eccentrically from aortic wall
- Bacterial aortitis most commonly caused by Salmonella or Staph aureus
- Syphilitic aortitis involves the ascending aorta but spares the aortic sinus
  - Ascending aorta most common location

Imaging Findings
General Features
- Best imaging clue: Rapidly growing saccular aneurysm arising eccentrically from aortic wall
CT Findings
- NECT
  - Bacterial aortitis is rarely calcified
  - Syphilitic aortitis shows curvilinear calcifications
- CECT: One or more saccular aneurysms arising form aortic wall
MR Findings
- T1WI
  - Periaortic low-signal intensity in absence of gadolinium (Gd)
  - Aortic and periaortic enhancement following Gd, especially evident on fat-suppressed images
- T2WI: Periaortic high-signal intensity on fat-suppressed T2WI
- Contrast enhanced MRA
  - One or more saccular aneurysms arising from aortic wall
  - Effacement of wall with possible leakage at rupture site
  - It is important to review MRA as well as delayed source images to identify areas of enhancement

Mycotic Aneurysm

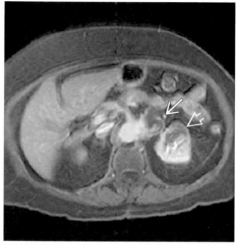

Delayed fat-suppressed T1 weighted gradient echo image in same patient as prior figure. Image demonstrates saccular aortic aneurysm (arrow) with associated renal abscess (open arrow).

<u>Imaging Recommendations</u>
- T1WI and T2WI MRI followed by contrast-enhanced MRA

Differential Diagnosis
<u>Atherosclerotic Aneurysm</u>
- Slow growing
- More often fusiform
- Often calcified

<u>Inflammatory Aneurysm</u>
- Distal aorta and iliac involvement
- Fusiform aneurysm
- Retro-peritoneal fibrosis

Pathology
<u>General</u>
- Normal aorta is resistant to infection
- Generally believed that mycotic aneurysm most often forms after diseased aorta is infected
- Etiology-Pathogenesis
  - Routes of infection
    - Most often caused by seeding of an existing lesion (atheroma or aneurysm) via the vasa vasorum
    - Direct extension from infection in vessel wall, i.e., bacterial endocarditis
    - Invasion of aortic wall by extravascular contiguous infection
    - Lymphatic spread
- Epidemiology
  - Increased risk in
    - IV drug abusers

Mycotic Aneurysm

- • Patients with history of bacterial endocarditis
- • Immunocompromised patients
- • Patients with vascular prostheses (valves, grafts)

Gross Pathologic or Surgical Features
- Bacterial aneurysm
  - o Non-calcified, saccular aneurysm
  - o Thinning of the aortic wall with periaortic inflammatory changes
- Syphilitic aneurysm
  - o Calcified lesion
  - o "Tree bark" appearance when atheroma develops in infected areas

Microscopic Features
- Loss of intima and destruction of internal elastic lamina
- Media shows varying degrees of destruction
- Bacteria present on histology

Staging Criteria
- Classification system
  - o Primary mycotic aneurysm arise from a distant, unknown, or remote source of infection
  - o Secondary mycotic aneurysm arise from specific source of infection
    - • Bacterial endocarditis (intravascular spread)
    - • Tuberculosis (contiguous spread)

Clinical Issues

Presentation
- Symptoms vary greatly
- Nonspecific findings
- Low-grade fever
- Localized pain
- Positive blood cultures

Natural History
- Nearly always fatal if untreated

Treatment
- Surgical resection/grafting following antibiotic therapy
- May need extra anatomic bypass grafting

Prognosis
- Acute rupture/hemorrhage seen in 75%
- Mortality rate estimated at 67%

Selected References
1. Gonda RL et al: Mycotic aneurysm of the aorta: Radiologic features. Radiology 168: 343-6, 1988
2. Vogelzang RL et al: Infected aortic aneurysm: CT appearance. JCAT 12(1): 109-12, 1988
3. Lande A et al: Aortitis: Pathologic, clinical, and radiographic review. Radiol Clin North Am 14: 219-40, 1976

Giant Cell Arteritis

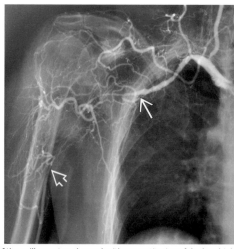

Occlusion of the axillary artery (arrow) with reconstitution of the brachial artery (open arrow) in a patient with giant cell arteritis. (Courtesy John Kaufman MD)

Key Facts
- Synonym: Temporal arteritis
- Definition: Arteritis involving segments of the media of large and medium sized arteries
- Classic imaging appearance: Alternating segments of smooth arterial narrowing and areas of mild dilatation
  - May be arterial occlusions
- Thoracic aortic aneurysm 17x more common than age-matched controls
- Abdominal aortic aneurysm 2x more common than age-matched controls
- Most common form of systemic vasculitis in adults
- Relationship with polymyalgia rheumatica
- If superficial temporal artery is involved, patient has pain over temporal artery and superficial temporal artery biopsy will make diagnosis
- Inflammatory disorder, often associated with constitutional symptoms

Imaging Findings
<u>General Features</u>
- Best imaging clue: Multiple arteries involved with segmental involvement of the arteries
- Narrowings tend to be smooth, long-segment tapered stenoses
- Arteries which may be involved include aorta, coronary, vertebral, distal subclavian, axillary, brachial, celiac, superior mesenteric, renal, iliac, femoral, ophthalmic, and retinal, the carotid is less commonly involved
<u>CT Findings</u>
- CECT
  - Aortic disease, aneurysmal dilatation as well as narrowing
  - Evidence of arterial narrowing better evaluated with 3D reconstruction
  - Thickening of aortic wall – evidence of inflammation

Giant Cell Arteritis

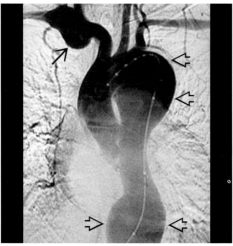

Giant cell arteritis with aneurysms involving the R subclavian/innominate (arrow), as well as two separate areas of descending aorta (open arrows). Abdominal aorta was involved as well. Aorta does not show evidence of atherosclerotic disease, and the aneurysms are smooth in appearance. (Courtesy Barry Katzen MD)

MR Findings
- Possible MR protocol: T2-weighted, pre- and post-intravenous contrast T1-weighted spin echo, MRA (2D time-of-flight) 3D angiography with contrast, STIR may be more sensitive to edema
- Findings similar to CT, but with additional imaging planes can see great vessel involvement with segmental arterial narrowing
- Evaluate for wall thickening, and wall enhancement with contrast

Ultrasound Findings
- Hypoechoic halo surrounding artery, reflecting edema of the wall
- May demonstrate narrowing particularly in the carotid arteries if they are involved

Angiography Findings
- Multiple segmental areas of narrowing in multiple vessels, predominately medium-sized vessels
- If the aorta is involved, then aneurysmal dilatation may be present

Imaging Recommendations
- MRI/MRA
- Angiography

Differential Diagnosis

Takayasu's Arteritis
- Also involves the large and medium sized arteries
- Tends to be in younger patients
- More likely to be female

Atherosclerotic Disease
- May be difficult to differentiate radiographically, but the clinical symptoms will help to make the diagnosis
- May not have the usual atherosclerotic risk factors

Giant Cell Arteritis

Vasculitis
- More likely to be in small and medium sized arteries
- Associated with collagen vascular disease
- Also commonly associated with constitutional symptoms

Pathology

General
- General Path Comments
  - Arteries affected by an inflammatory infiltrate associated with marked disruption of the internal elastic lamina
  - Thoracic aortic aneurysms and dissection of the aorta are important late complications of giant cell arteritis
  - Thoracic aortic aneurysm 17 times more common in giant cell arteritis
- Etiology-Pathogenesis
  - Parvovirus or parainfluenza virus may have a role
  - T lymphocytes seem to be key players
  - Macrophages appear to be activated by the T cells and then differentiate to cause damage by a variety of mechanisms
  - Clinical subsets result from variable cytokine expression
- Epidemiology
  - Occurs most frequently in the fifth and sixth decades
  - Occurs twice as often in women compared to men

Microscopic Features
- Vasculitis characterized by a predominance of mononuclear cell infiltrates or granulomatous inflammation, usually with multinucleated giant cells at junction between the intima and media

Clinical Issues

Presentation
- Clinical symptoms include: Headache, malaise, fever, jaw claudication, polymyalgia rheumatica, and visual symptoms including blindness, claudication of arms or less commonly legs
- Marked elevation in the erythrocyte sedimentation rate
- Biopsy of the superficial temporal artery will make diagnosis

Treatment
- Responds rapidly to corticosteroid treatment
- May also be treated with methotrexate and steroids
- Patients 2-5 times more likely to develop complications of steroid treatment - diabetes, osteoporosis

Prognosis
- Despite response to steroid therapy, arteries may have residual narrowing

Selected References
1.   Levine SM et al: Giant cell arteritis. Curr Opin Rheumatol 14: 3-10, 2002
2.   Salvarani C et al: Polymyalgia rheumatica and giant-cell arteritis. NEJM 347: 261-71, 2002
3.   Atalay MK et al: Magnetic resonance imaging of large vessel vasculitis. Curr Opin Rheumatol 13: 41-7, 2001

Aortic Dissection

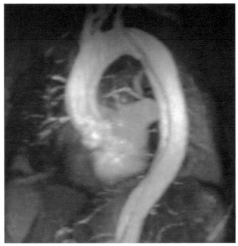

MRA of Type B dissection. Dissection flap extends from just distal to the origin of the left subclavian artery into abdomen. MRI/MRA allows for rotation of the image in multiple orientations to delineate the extent of dissection and the involvement of branch vessels. (Courtesy Gabrella Iussiah MD)

Key Facts
- Definition: A spectrum of pathology in which blood enters the media of the aortic wall and splits it in a longitudinal fashion
  - Type A (60%): Involves at least ascending aorta; surgical treatment
  - Type B (40%): Limited to descending aorta; medical treatment
- Classic imaging appearance: "Double barrel" aorta with an interposed intimal flap
- Additional imaging appearance
  - Extensive longitudinal extent (> 6 cm), calcification appears displaced into aorta; great vessels, celiac, renal artery, SMA, iliac artery involvement
- Abnormal CXR (25% are normal) is nonspecific

Imaging Findings
General Features
- Best imaging clue: Intimal flap and 2 lumens
CT Findings
- Intimal flap is seen as linear filling defect within aortic lumen
- Evaluate thrombosed false channels, periaortic hematoma and pericardial/ pleural blood, and isolated aortic wall hematoma
MR Findings
- Conventional spin echo: Excellent for intimal flap and wall hematoma
- Phase contrast gradient echo detects differential flow velocities in true and false lumens
- Evaluate extent of dissection, site of entry tear, arch vessels involvement, renal artery involvement, mesenteric and pelvic artery involvement
TEE Findings
- Most important finding: Presence of an undulating intimal flap within the aortic lumen that differentiates a false lumen from a true lumen

Aortic Dissection

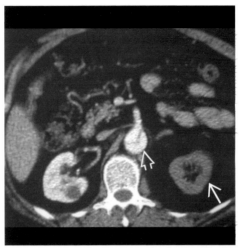

CT of type B dissection. Dissection flap seen extending into the abdominal aorta (open arrow). Note the lack of perfusion of the left kidney (arrow). This indicates involvement of the left renal artery by the dissection with compromise of the blood flow to the kidney.

- Identify entry site, presence of thrombus in false lumen, abnormal flow characteristics, involvement of coronary and arch vessels, pericardial effusion, and aortic valve regurgitation

Angiography Findings
- Evaluate extent of dissection, site of intimal tears, aortic valve regurgitation, coronary artery involvement, and filling of branch vessels

Imaging Recommendations
- CT scan highly accurate for diagnosis, slightly less accurate for dissection of the ascending aorta
- MRI well suited for evaluation of patients with previous aortic disease
- TEE ideal for use in most patients, including relatively unstable ones
  - Highly dependent on investigator's experience
  - Cannot be used on patients with esophageal varicosities or stenosis

Differential Diagnosis

Thrombosed Aneurysm
- Calcification outside aortic shadow
- Large aorta and aortic lumen size
- Branches involved: Lumbars, inferior mesenteric artery (IMA)

Aortic Wall Hematoma
- Hemorrhage within wall with no identifiable intimal flap or false lumen
- Caused by bleeding from vasa vasorum into the media
- Imaging: Hyperdense aortic wall

Penetrating Aortic Ulcer
- Tear of aortic wall in a region of ulcerated atherosclerotic plaque
- Most common in descending aorta
- Clinical symptoms may mimic aortic dissection

Aortic Dissection

Pathology

<u>General</u>
- General Path Comments
  - Spontaneous dissections almost exclusively originate in the thoracic aorta and secondarily involve the abdominal aorta by extension
  - Smooth muscle myosin heavy chain marker helpful in diagnosis
- Etiology-Pathogenesis
  - Medial degeneration is a pathologic finding associated with many diseases that predispose to dissection
    - Hypertension, structural collagen disorder (Marfan's, Ehlers-Danlos), congenital (aortic coarctation, bicuspid or unicuspid valve), pregnancy, collagen vascular disease (very uncommon)
- Epidemiology
  - Peak age: 50-70
  - Men > women (3:1)
  - History of hypertension obtained in 65% of cases

Clinical Issues

<u>Presentation</u>
- Sharp, tearing chest pain or back pain (80-90%)
- Aortic insufficiency
- Blood pressure discrepancies between extremities
- Neurologic defects
- Ischemic extremity
- Silent dissections are very rare

<u>Natural History</u>
- Poorly understood
- Dissection propagates in the media at varying depths until a rupture occurs either into lumen of the aorta, or out through adventitia, causing death

<u>Treatment</u>
- Type A: Requires surgery because of involvement of aortic root
  - Pericardial tamponade, coronary artery occlusion, aortic insufficiency
- Type B: Medical control of hypertension is standard therapy
  - Surgery in complicated cases
    - Mesenteric, renal, extremity ischemia; rupture, aneurysmal enlargement of false lumen
- Percutaneous fenestration of luminal flap helpful for nonsurgical patients
- Aortic stent grafting may be option for nonsurgical patients

<u>Prognosis</u>
- 21% patients die before hospital admission
- < 10% of untreated patients with Type A live 1 year
- Surgical long-term survival approaching 60% with surgical mortality 5-10%

Selected References
1. Khan IA et al: Clinical, diagnostic, and management perspectives of aortic dissection. Chest 122 (1): 311-28, 2002
2. Hartnell GG: Imaging of aortic aneurysms and dissection: CT and MRI. J Thorac Imaging 16: 35-46, 2001
3. Weissleder R et al: Primer of Diagnostic Imaging. 2nd ed, 614-7, 1997

Traumatic Aortic Laceration

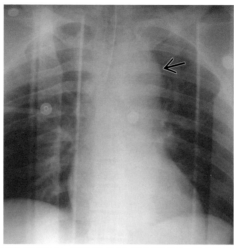

Traumatic aortic laceration. AP chest x-ray demonstrates widening of the superior mediastinum, rightward tracheal deviation and indistinct aortic knob (arrow). Patient involved in high-speed motor vehicle accident. (Courtesy Don Yandow MD)

Key Facts
- Synonyms: Aortic pseudoaneurysm, aortic rupture, traumatic aortic aneurysm, aortic transection
- Definition: Aortic laceration or rupture secondary to sudden horizontal (MVA) or vertical (fall from great height) deceleration injury of the thorax
- Classic imaging appearance
  - Mediastinal widening
  - Localized saccular outpouching of aorta
- Location
  - 88% aortic isthmus
  - 4.5% aortic arch with avulsion of brachiocephalic trunk
  - 2% descending thoracic aorta
  - 1% ascending aorta immediately above aortic valve

Imaging Findings
Chest Radiography Findings
- Mediastinal widening > 8 cm (75%)
- Indistinct aortic outline (75% at arch, 12% at descending)
- Esophageal/nasogastric tube deviation to right (67%)
- Tracheal displacement to right (61%)
- Inferior displacement of left mainstem bronchus (53%)
- Apical pleural cap (37%)
- First or second rib fracture (17%)
CT Findings
- NECT
  - 55% sensitive, 65% specific
  - Obliteration of aortic-fat interface with increased attenuation suggesting mediastinal hemorrhage
- CECT
  - Negative CT has nearly 100% negative predictive value

Traumatic Aortic Laceration

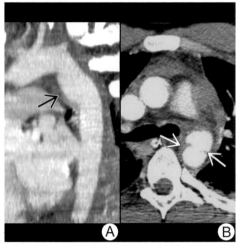

Traumatic aortic laceration. (A) Reformatted image and (B) axial image from contrast-enhanced CT demonstrates aortic pseudoaneurysm (black arrow) with focal intimal disruption (white arrows) and periaortic edema and hemorrhage. (Courtesy Don Yandow MD)

- o Abrupt change of aortic contour
- o Extravasation of contrast
- o Intimal flap
- o Pseudocoarctation secondary to diminished caliber descending aorta
- o May require multiplanar reformatting
  - ▪ Acquire using thin sections for CTA
  - ▪ Use rapid IV contrast bolus (2-5 cc/sec for 100-150 cc)

MR Findings
- Generally not used in acute setting
- MR angiography may be used for equivocal cases

Echocardiography Findings
- Newer techniques in transesophageal echocardiogram (TEE) are accurate
  - o Proximal ascending and descending aorta may be seen
  - o May be performed at bedside

Angiography Findings
- Classically was gold standard but recent advances in CTA have led to limited role of routine angiography
- Rupture with extravasation of contrast material
- Intimal flap (5-10%)
- Posttraumatic dissection (11%)
- Technique
  - o At least two views optimal, prefer 45° lateral anterior oblique (LAO), AP and lateral view
  - o Rate 30 cc/sec for total volume 60 cc
  - o Consider brachial approach if possible

Imaging Recommendations
- Initial study chest x-ray then consider CECT unless urgent surgery required due to unstable clinical status

Traumatic Aortic Laceration

Differential Diagnosis
Ductus Diverticulum
- Located at aortic isthmus in 10% of normal population
- Smooth contour with obtuse margin

Penetrating Atherosclerotic Ulcer
- Location usually not at inner aspect of aortic isthmus
- Look for associated calcified atherosclerotic plaque

Pathology
General
- General path comments
  - Shear stress at points of maximal fixation of aorta
  - Laceration most often transverse
  - All layers of aortic wall involved in only 40%
- Epidemiology
  - Fall from great heights
  - Rapid deceleration

Gross Pathologic or Surgical Features
- Intimal tear with mediastinal hematoma

Clinical Issues
Presentation
- Exsanguination before reaching hospital (85% of total)
- Chest pain
- Dyspnea
- Dysphagia
- Hypertension in upper extremities secondary to traumatic coarctation
- Bilateral femoral pulse deficits
- Systolic murmur in second left parasternal interface

Natural History
- 15-20% initial survival rate
- May develop chronic posttraumatic pseudoaneurysm
  - Defined as present > 3 months
  - Incidence: 2-5% patients surviving aortic transection > 24-48 hr
  - Most commonly at level of ligamentum arteriosum
- Incomplete rupture (15% of total)
  - Progression to complete rupture within 24 hours (50%)
  - False aneurysm formation (40-60%)

Treatment
- Surgical repair
  - Left thoracotomy with placement of interposition graft or primary anastomosis

Prognosis
- With surgery 60-70% survival rate
- Without intervention
  - 80% death within 1 hour
  - 85% death within 24 hours
  - 98% death within 10 weeks

Selected References
1. Dahnert WF: Radiology review manual 4th Ed, Lippincott Williams & Wilkins, Philadelphia, 513-4, 1999
2. Randall PA et al: Aneurysms of the thoracic aorta in Abrams' angiography. 4th Ed., 477-83, 1997
3. Kadir S: Diagnostic angiography, W. B. Saunders, Philadelphia, 149-56, 1986

Aortic Ulceration

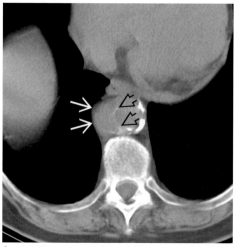

Ulceration of aorta. Even on non-enhanced CT scan, one should be suspicious of ulcer. Bulging out of the aortic wall (arrows) with more than normal caliber above and below. Also note the break in the calcification (open arrows). (Courtesy John Kaufman MD)

Key Facts

- Synonyms: Penetrating aortic ulcer, penetrating atherosclerotic ulcer
- Definition: An ulcerating atherosclerotic lesion that penetrates the elastic lamina and is associated with hematoma formation within the media of aortic wall
- Classic imaging appearance: Focal involvement of the aorta with adjacent subintimal hematoma located beneath the calcified and inwardly displaced intima in the middle or distal third of the thoracic aorta
- Often associated with thickening or enhancement of the aortic wall
- Usually with evidence of severe atherosclerosis of the surrounding aorta
- Imaging may reveal pleural/pericardial fluid, mediastinal hematoma, or pseudoaneurysm

Imaging Findings

General Features
- Best imaging clue: Crater-like outpouching of the lumen, thickened aortic wall, and inward displacement of the calcified intima by the intramural hematoma

Chest Radiography Findings
- Generally no findings, might see a focal widening of the descending thoracic aorta

CT Findings
- Focal ulceration of the aortic wall
- Inward displacement of intima, intima commonly calcified
- Reconstructions may be helpful to delineate ulcer and mural abnormalities

MR Findings
- Superior to CT in differentiating acute intramural hematoma from atherosclerotic plaque and chronic intraluminal thrombus
- Gadolinium enhancement improves evaluation

Aortic Ulceration

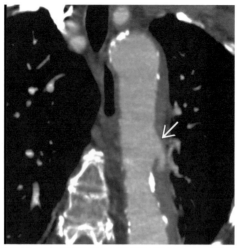

Contrast enhanced, CT reconstruction of the thoracic aorta demonstrating an ulcer (arrow) protruding from the lateral wall of the aorta. Thickening of the aortic wall is also present. (Courtesy Claude Sirlin MD)

- Focal ulcerated contrast collection in the aortic wall
- Thickening of the aortic wall

Transesophageal Echocardiography
- Focal outpouching in atherosclerotic wall that occurs in middle to distal portion of the descending thoracic aorta

Angiography
- Ulcerated lesion in the descending thoracic aorta
- Intravascular ultrasound can be used to characterize plaque components

Imaging Recommendations
- Spiral CECT recommended because of shorter examination time
- Gadolinium MRI is the modality of choice if iodinated contrast material is contraindicated

Differential Diagnosis

Aortic Dissection
- Presence of smooth intimal flap that extends across the aorta to create a false lumen
- Length often extensive
- May involve ascending aorta

Intramural Hematoma
- Concentrically located collection of blood within the media of aortic wall
- No intimal flap or ulcer crater

Mycotic Aneurysm
- More inflammatory appearance of the ulcer
- Fever, elevated WBC, positive blood cultures suggest diagnosis

Pseudoaneurysm
- Usually in areas where typically trauma involves the aorta; ligamentum arteriosum, diaphragmatic hiatus, root of aorta
- Clinical history of trauma

Aortic Ulceration

Pathology

General

- General Path Comments
  - Location
    - Most commonly mid and distal descending thoracic aorta
    - Can occur at any point along the length of aorta
  - Size
    - Diameter 5-25 mm
    - Depth 4-30 mm
  - Strong association with concomitant or previously treated aneurysms at other sites
- Etiology-Pathogenesis
  - Progression of atherosclerosis
    - Ulcer penetrates through elastic lamina and extends into media
    - Media exposed to pulsatile blood flow, resulting in intramural hematoma and variable degree of dissection
- Epidemiology
  - True incidence not known
  - Risk factors: Hypertension, advanced atherosclerosis
  - Predominant age: Elderly
  - Predominant sex: Male > female

Microscopic Features

- Extensive surrounding atherosclerosis
- Ulcer penetrates internal elastic lamina and extends into media

Clinical Issues

Presentation

- Often asymptomatic, patient may have hypertension, hyperlipidemia
- Symptoms
  - Severe chest/ back pain
  - Embolization of atheroma (uncommon)

Natural History

- May progress to dissection
- Possibility of aortic dilation and aneurysm formation

Treatment

- Medical therapy (antihypertensive) and close monitoring if pain resolves and there is no evidence of deterioration
- Surgical intervention indications
  - Persistent or recurring pain, hemodynamic instability, rapidly expanding aortic diameter, embolization

Prognosis

- Little is known about natural history
- Prevalence of critical cases of symptomatic penetrating ulcer is higher than that of classical aortic dissection

Selected References
1. Sueyoshi E et al: New development of an ulcerlike projection in aortic intramural hematoma: CT evaluation. Radiology 224: 536-41, 2002
2. Troxler M et al: Penetrating atherosclerotic ulcers of the aorta. Br J of Surg 88: 1169-77, 2001
3. Hayashi H et al: Penetrating atherosclerotic ulcer of the aorta: Imaging features and disease concept. Radiographics 20: 995-1005, 2000

Pulmonary Embolism (PE)

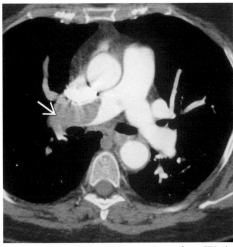

Massive pulmonary embolism (PE). Axial source image form CTA shows large PE occluding the right pulmonary artery (arrow).

Key Facts
- Common disease, any hospitalized patient at risk
- Chest radiograph nonspecific, 10% normal
- Pulmonary infarcts uncommon, may be any shape or size
- CT angiography examination of choice, highly sensitive and specific
- Outcomes for negative CT angiograms good (< 1% embolic rate)
- Pulmonary angiography rarely performed

Imaging Findings
Chest Radiography Findings
- 10% normal
- Most abnormalities nonspecific
- Vascular alteration
  - Focal enlargement of central pulmonary artery (knuckle sign)
    - Commonly right interlobar pulmonary artery
    - Due to physical presence of clot
  - Focal oligemia (Westermark sign)
    - Due to vascular obstruction
- Pulmonary infarct
  - < 10% embolic episodes result in infarction
  - Infarction more common in those with underlying cardiopulmonary disease
  - May develop immediately or delayed 2-3 days following embolus
  - Any size or shape
    - Usually peripheral or in lower lung zones
    - Often associated with small pleural effusion
  - Evolution
    - Initially ill defined, over time become sharply defined resolution
    - 50% clear completely usually within 3 weeks

Pulmonary Embolism (PE)

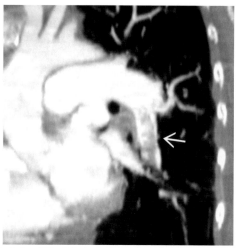

Pulmonary embolism (PE). Multiplanar reformation of left lower lobe pulmonary artery shows filling defect from partially occlusive acute PE (arrow).

- Others leave linear scars (Fleischner lines)
  - Hampton's hump
    - Peripheral wedge-shaped opacity with rounded apex pointing toward the hilum
  - Infarcts "melt"
    - Maintain their initial shape and shrink over time
    - Pneumonia and edema generally "fade" away

V/Q Scanning Findings
- Indirect indicator of clot, does not directly visualize the clot
- High sensitivity but poor specificity
  - Normal perfusion scan excludes embolus
- Interobserver agreement poor for low and indeterminate V/Q category (30%)

CT Findings
- Spiral or electron beam CT revolutionized diagnosis of PE
- Directly visualizes clot in central pulmonary artery
- High sensitivity and specificity (> 90%)
- Pitfalls
  - Poor bolus
  - Hilar lymph nodes
  - Breathing artifacts
  - May miss subsegmental emboli
  - Oblique arteries may require oblique reconstructions to adequately visualize
- High observer agreement
- Can be combined with scanning pelvis and thighs for thromboembolic disease
- Outcomes of negative CT angiograms good
  - Fatal embolism 0-0.7%

Pulmonary Embolism (PE)

Pulmonary Angiography Findings
- Now primarily performed in clinical practice if thrombolysis Rx planned
- Considered gold standard
  - 25% false negative for small subsegmental emboli
- Interobserver agreement poor for subsegmental emboli (> 30%)

Differential Diagnosis
Pneumonia
- Common in critically ill, nonspecific opacities must consider embolus
Atelectasis
- Common in critically ill, nonspecific opacities must consider embolus

Pathology
General
- Pulmonary emboli end result of thrombosis in peripheral veins generally of the lower extremities
- Epidemiology
  - Considered 3rd most common cause of death
  - Any hospitalized patient at risk for emboli, other risk factors
    - Trauma
    - Surgery
    - Obesity
    - Pregnancy, birth control pills
    - Malignancy
    - Myocardial infarction
    - Antithrombin-III deficiency
Gross Pathologic or Surgical Features
- Hemodynamic consequences
  - > 50% reduction vascular bed leads to pulmonary hypertension and right heart failure
- Deep venous clot fragments in right heart, an average of 8 vessels embolized

Clinical Issues
Presentation
- No telltale signs, symptoms, or laboratory studies that strongly suggest PE
Treatment
- Anticoagulation and fibrinolysis
  - Hemorrhage complications in 2–15%
- IVC filter if contraindications to drug therapy
Prognosis
- Good with appropriate therapy, must maintain high index of suspicion as mortality for untreated disease is 20%
- Outcomes for untreated subsegmental emboli unknown
  - Outcome following negative pulmonary angiograms or CT is good

Selected References
1. Elliott CG et al: Chest radiographs in acute pulmonary embolism: Results from the international cooperative pulmonary embolism registry. Chest 118: 33-8, 2000
2. Remy-Jardin M et al: Spiral CT angiography of the pulmonary circulation. Radiology 212: 615-36, 1999

Hereditary Hemorrhagic Telangiectasia

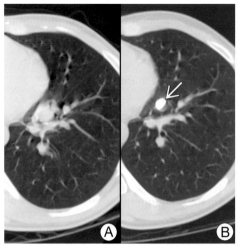

(A) Screening NECT scan of the lung in a patient with know HHT revealed a large pulmonary AVM. (B) Post-embolization study shows successful endovascular occlusion of the AVM (arrow). (Courtesy Frank J Miller MD)

Key Facts
- Synonyms: HHT, Osler-Weber-Rendu (Rendu-Osler-Weber) syndrome
- Definition: Autosomal dominant disorder with mucocutaneous and visceral telangiectasias +/- AVFs in brain, lungs, GI tract (including liver)
- Classic imaging appearance: Multiple intracranial AVMs, visceral AVMs
- Most common presentation = epistaxis
- Neurologic symptoms common
  - o Parenchymal or SAH with brain AVM
  - o TIA, stroke, abscess as complications of pulmonary AVMs

Imaging Findings
General Features
- Best imaging clue: Multiple pulmonary (pAVM) or cerebral (cAVM) arteriovenous malformations in patient with recurrent epistaxis
CT Findings
- NECT
  - o Lung: High resolution NON CONTRAST multislice CT shows well-delineated vascular mass(es), usually in lower lobes
  - o Brain
    - ▪ AVM = Isodense serpentine vessels
    - ▪ Abscess = Low density mass with iso-/hyperdense rim
- CECT: Strong, uniform, well-delineated intravascular enhancement
MR Findings (Vary with Flow Rate, Direction, Presence of Hemorrhage)
- T1WI: "Flow voids" common, variable hemorrhage
- T2WI: "Flow voids"
- Other Sequences: GRE demonstrates flow in cAVMs
Other Modality Findings
- Angiography (DSA, MRA, CTA) demonstrates AVMs/AVFs in affected organs

Hereditary Hemorrhagic Telangiectasia

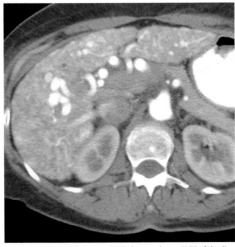

Axial CECT scan in a patient with known HHT shows a large AVM of the liver. (Courtesy Frank J Miller MD)

<u>Imaging Recommendations</u>
- Multislice CT of lungs, liver
- MR, MRA of brain

Differential Diagnosis
<u>Multiple Intracranial AVMs</u>
- Rare; 50% not associated with HHT

Pathology
<u>General</u>
- General Path Comments
  - Abnormalities of vascular structure account for all recognized phenotypic manifestations of HHT
- Genetics
  - Autosomal dominant inheritance
  - HHT associated with two known mutations
    - Type 1 HHT: Endoglin gene (chromosome 9q33-q34) mutation
    - Type 2 HHT: ALK-1 gene mutation
    - Third as yet unidentified group
  - Missense, nonsense, frameshift, deletion mutations have been identified
- Etiology-Pathogenesis
  - Abnormal intracellular signal transduction during angiogenesis
  - Abnormalities of transforming growth factor-beta (TGF-β) receptors
- Epidemiology
  - Rare; 1/15,000-20,000 births
  - 70% of patients with pAVMs have HHT
  - 5-15% of people with HHT have pAVMs
  - At least 50% of patients with multiple cAVMs have HHT
  - 5-13% of patients with HHT have cAVMs
  - 2- 17% have hepatic AVMs (depends on kindred)

Hereditary Hemorrhagic Telangiectasia

<u>Gross Pathologic or Surgical Features</u>
- Multiple telangiectasias of mucosa, dermis almost universal
- AVMs, AVFs appear in only certain forms of HHT
  - Most pAVMs are actually AVFs (direct connection between pulmonary artery and vein through thin-walled aneurysm)
  - Hepatic AV shunts less common, often numerous

<u>Microscopic Features</u>
- Smallest telangiectasias = focal dilatations of post-capillary venules
- Larger lesions extend through entire dermis, often connect directly to dilated arterioles

<u>Staging or Grading Criteria</u>
- Most cAVMs in HHT are low-grade (Spetzler - Martin I or II)

Clinical Issues
<u>Presentation</u>
- Most common = recurrent epistaxis from nasal mucosal telangiectasias
  - Begins by age 10
- Skin lesions appear later (most by 40y)
- Pulmonary AVMs cause R/L shunts, dyspnea, cyanosis, fatigue, polycythemia; may be complicated by cerebral emboli/abscess

<u>Natural History</u>
- Epistaxis increases in frequency, severity
- Cerebral AVMs in HHT have lower bleeding risk than sporadic AVMs; rare cases may regress spontaneously

<u>Treatment</u>
- Surgical: No longer indicated because of excellent results with embolization for pAVMs
- Options: Embolotherapy/stereotaxic radiosurgery for cAVMs
- Mucosal telangiectasias (nose, GI tract) can be treated with laser coagulation
- Prophylactic antibiotics prior to all dental work if pAVM present
- I.V. iron useful when oral iron fails to keep stores at satisfactory level

<u>Prognosis</u>
- Epistaxis begins by age 10y, most have by age 21y
- Can be severe, exsanguinating
- Significant lifetime risk of brain abscess or stroke if pAVM present
- Heart failure a poor prognoses in patients with hepatic AVM
- GI bleeding also limits lifespan when occurs under age 50; many require multiple transfusions and endoscopies

Selected References
1. Azuma H: Genetic and molecular pathogenesis of hereditary hemorrhagic telangiectasia. J Med Invest 47: 81-90, 2000
2. McDonald JE et al: Clinical manifestations in a large hereditary hemorrhagic telangiectasia type 2 indred. Am J Med Genet 93: 320-7, 2000
3. Guttmacher AE et al: Hereditary hemorrhagic telangiectasia. NEJM 333: 918-24, 1995

PocketRadiologist™
Vascular
Top 100 Diagnoses

ABDOMINAL

Infected Aortic Graft

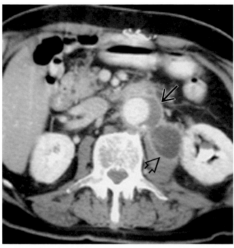

Patient had aortic graft replacement 5 years previously. Now presents with fever and left back pain. Fluid collection around graft with enhancing rim (arrow). The fluid extends into the psoas muscle on the left (open arrow) also with enhancement. (Courtesy Pauline Chu MD)

Key Facts
- Synonym: Postoperative graft infection
- Definition: Infection of aortic prosthetic graft
- Classic imaging appearance: Perigraft fluid, soft-tissue density, or ectopic gas beyond four weeks after surgery
- Other key facts
  - Incidence = 1-6% of all postoperative aortic graft patients
  - Serious complication with mortality rates of 25-75%
  - Graft infection is 3x more common if aorta is ruptured preoperatively
  - Most common organism is staphylococcus epidermis
  - Hematoma after graft placement should resolve within 3 months
  - Aortic enteric fistula is a subset of aortic graft infections

Imaging Findings
General Features
- Best imaging clue: Perigraft fluid, soft-tissue mass, increasing or persisting months after graft placement
- Perigraft air more prevalent with an aortoenteric fistula
CT Findings
- NECT: Perigraft fluid, perigraft soft tissue density
  - Ectopic perigraft gas represents aortoenteric fistula
- CECT
  - Perigraft inflammatory enhancement
  - Leakage of contrast into pseudoaneurysm, most pseudoaneurysms not infected
MR Findings
- T1WI: Perigraft soft-tissue mass, fluid collection low signal
- T2WI: Perigraft fluid collection high signal intensity
- Contrast-enhanced MR
  - Contrast-enhancement of perigraft inflammatory mass

Infected Aortic Graft

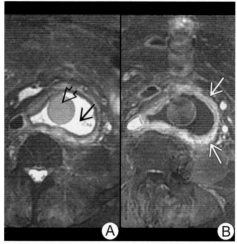

Graft infection (A) T2WI shows high-signal fluid (black arrow) around aortic graft (open arrow), a non-specific finding early after graft placement. (B) T1WI post-contrast shows marked enhancement of aortic wall due to infection (arrows). (Courtesy Thomas M Grist MD)

   o Look for evidence of inflammatory changes in psoas muscles
Other Modality Findings
- Ultrasound not very helpful in evaluating aortic graft infection
- Nuclear medicine: Indium-111 labeled white blood cell, Gallium scans
- Angiography: Only for preoperative road map of arteries for extraanatomic grafting
Imaging Recommendations
- Unenhanced and enhanced CT as first imaging test
- In-111 labeled WBC scan important test if CT ambiguous
- MRA, CTA, or conventional angiography is very helpful to establish the status of vessels distal to the graft, for possible secondary repair (i.e., axillary-femoral bypass procedure)

Differential Diagnosis
Anastomotic Pseudoaneurysm
- Caused by failure of graft repair at suture line, placing excessive tension on anastomosis
- Anastomotic pseudoaneurysms may result as a secondary complication of infection of graft
Aortoenteric Fistula
- Breakdown of graft repair with erosion of aortic contents into bowel
- Duodenum is most common location of aortoenteric fistula
Normal Postoperative Resolution of Perigraft Hematoma
- Complete resolution of hematomas should occur within 3 months
- Ectopic gas in early postoperative period is suspicious but not diagnostic, gas should be resorbed in 3-4 weeks

Infected Aortic Graft

Pathology
Cenital
- Most infections are believed to be a result of contamination from the abdominal incision
- Hematogenous seeding secondary to bacteremia may be a cause of late graft infection
- Etiology-Pathogenesis
  - Most common organism is staphylococcus epidermidis
    - Produces a slime that adheres to the graft and protects organism from host and from antibiotics, very difficult to eradicate
  - Many of organisms are fastidious and may require 14 days to culture

Clinical Issues
Presentation
- Signs and symptoms are not specific
  - Fever
  - Malaise
  - Back or abdominal pain
  - Gastrointestinal bleeding
  - Elevated sedimentation rate
  - Palpable mass
  - Draining sinus
- Patients may present days to years following surgery
Treatment
- Antibiotic therapy often not curative
- Percutaneous aspiration of fluid around graft
  - Diagnostic, obtain fluid for microbiology examination
  - Occasionally therapeutic
  - Installation of thrombolytics has been tried to help clear staph epidermidis. infection
- Graft excision and placement of extraanatomic bypass
  - Occasionally autogenous vein in situ, or very rarely rifampin-bonded prosthesis in situ
Prognosis
- High morbidity and mortality associated with operative repair of infected graft

Selected References
1. Orton DF et al: Aortic prosthetic graft infections: Radiologic manifestations and implications for management. Radiographics 20: 977-93, 2000
2. Modrall JG et al: The role of imaging techniques in evaluating possible graft infections. Semin Vasc Surg 12: 339-47, 1999
3. Valentine RJ: Diagnosis and management of aortic graft infection. Semin Vasc Surg 14: 292-301, 2001

Aortic Aneurysm

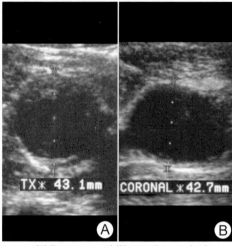

Aortic Aneurysm. (A) Transverse, and (B) coronal grayscale ultrasound images.

Key Facts
- Definition: Dilatation of the aorta (Ao) ≥ 1.5 times the normal diameter (5 cm ascending Ao, 4 cm arch/thoracic Ao, 3 cm distal abdominal Ao)
- May occur any part of Ao, most common distal abdominal Ao
- Degenerative, posttraumatic or post-infectious etiology

Imaging Findings
General Features
- Best imaging clue: Focal or diffuse Ao dilatation
- Aneurysm (AN) shape related to cause
  - Fusiform and concentric: Usually degenerative (age-related AN)
  - Focal and eccentric: Suggests mycotic or posttraumatic origin
- Always measure AN outer-to-outer
CT/MR Findings
- IV contrast-enhanced studies preferred, look for
  - Diameter and linear extent of AN
  - Relationship of AN to major Ao branches
  - Amount of intraluminal thrombus
  - Extravasation due to leak/rupture
  - Inflammatory changes in fat surrounding Ao
- CT survey: 5 mm slices, area of interest (thorax or abdomen)
- CT surgical planning: 3 mm slices entire AN and adjacent normal Ao, 1 mm overlap for reconstruction
- Leaking/ruptured AN
  - Subtle: Indistinct region (hematoma) or localized contrast accumulation adjacent to AN, especially between AN and spine
  - Obvious
    - Hematoma adjacent to/surrounding AN
    - Hematoma in mediastinum/retroperitoneum
    - Blood in pleural/peritoneal spaces
  - Protocol for possible Ao AN rupture
    - Unstable patient, diagnosis likely – direct to surgery

Aortic Aneurysm

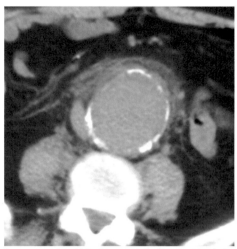

Mycotic aortic aneurysm (aortitis). CT scan at the iliac crest level shows an aortic aneurysm of about 6 cm diameter. Note thickened, indistinct appearance of aneurysm wall reflecting inflammation. Aortitis developed about 10 days after cardiac catheterization.

- Stable patient – CT (preferably with IV contrast)

Ultrasound Findings
- Defines size and extent of AN
- Best method for following AN for potential growth

Plain Chest and Abdominal Radiographs
- Enlarged Ao shadow or splayed calcified Ao walls
- Rounded, calcified mass at Ao arch, (chronic pseudoaneurysm)

Angiography Findings
- Focal or fusiform dilatation of Ao lumen
- Evaluate relationship of AN to branch vessels and assess for associated disease

Imaging Recommendations
- Ultrasound to detect, size and follow abdominal Ao ANs
- Contrast CT
  - To diagnose thoracic AN
  - For all surgical planning
  - For possible aneurysm leak
- Contrast MRI – substituted for CT with renal insufficiency

Differential Diagnosis

Aortic Dissection
- Separation of the layers of the aortic wall by entry of blood through a rent in the intima
- Usual causes
  - Age-related degeneration of the media layer
  - Inherited disorder of connective tissue (e.g. Ehlers-Danlos syndrome)

Penetrating Atherosclerotic Ulcer
- Focal AN or dissection at ulcerated atherosclerotic plaque (usually in thoracic Ao)

Aortic Aneurysm

Pathology
Genereal

- True AN: Wall layers intact but stretched
- Pseudoaneurysm: Wall layers penetrated
- Etiology-Pathogenesis
  - Age-related deterioration of the elastic media of the Ao
    - Most common cause
    - Associated with atherosclerosis, but not caused by atherosclerosis
  - Inherited weakness of arterial wall
    - Ehlers-Danlos syndrome, Marfan syndrome, fibromuscular dysplasia
  - Infection
    - Mycotic AN: De novo infection of the Ao wall **causing** AN
    - Infected AN: **Secondary** infection of a pre-existing Ao AN
  - Trauma
    - Rent in Ao wall with contained leak (pseudoaneurysm)
    - Subsequently ensconced with fibrous tissue, peripheral Ca++
    - Chronic Ao pseudoaneurysm = persistent rupture risk
- Epidemiology
  - Age-related ANs
    - More common in men than women
    - Most common 7th decade and beyond
    - Usually at the distal end of the abdominal Ao
    - Frequently associated iliac artery AN
  - Genetic-induced ANs present in young adulthood or beyond

Gross Pathology

- Fusiform ANs, particularly in distal Ao, contain variable amount of mural thrombus
  - Inner layer, more recently formed, non-organized thrombus
  - Outer layers, loose cellular matrix, no structural support
  - May embolize to extremities causing arterial occlusion

Clinical Issues
Presentation

- Usually asymptomatic, diagnosis on PE or imaging studies
- First sign may be catastrophic rupture
- Symptoms: Chest, back or abdominal pain, distal embolization
- Aortic valvular insufficiency, with ascending Ao ANs

Natural History

- Distal aortic ANs enlarge progressively at variable rate
  - Repair warranted: 5 cm diameter, rapid enlargement
- Mycotic/infected ANs: High short-term rupture risk
- Pseudoaneurysm: High short- and long-term rupture risk

Treatment

- Thoracic: Prosthetic graft repair (high risk surgery)
- Abdominal: Prosthetic graft (good outcome, durable) or endoluminal stent graft (presently reserved for poor surgical risk)

Selected References
1. Marin ML et al: Endovascular grafts. Semin Vasc Surg 12: 64-73,1999
2. Rutherford RB: Abdominal aortic aneurysms: New approaches to a continuing problem. Seminars in Vascular Surgery 8: 83-167, 1995
3. Cramer MM: Color flow duplex examination of the abdominal aorta. J Vasc Tech 19: 249-60, 1995

AAA with Rupture

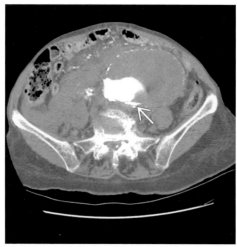

Large abdominal aneurysm with free fluid in the abdomen. Contrast collection extending away from the main opacified lumen (arrow). Fluid in abdomen measured 43-53 Hounsfield units consistent with bleeding. Patient with abdominal pain.

Key Facts
- Definition: Break in the wall of an abdominal aortic aneurysm (AAA)
- Classic imaging appearance
- Acute: Crescentic collection of contrast in the midst of extensive blood in the mesentery and retroperitoneum
- Chronic: Hematoma adjacent to the aneurysm
- In a chronic contained rupture (pseudoaneurysm) the leak is contained by the retroperitoneal soft tissues

Imaging Findings
General Features
- Best imaging clue (CT)
  - Acute: Obscuration or anterior displacement of the aneurysm by an irregular high-density mass into one or both perirenal spaces, and less commonly pararenal spaces
  - Chronic
    - Noncontrast: Well-defined mass extending from aorta with an attenuation value similar to or lower than that of the native aorta
    - Postcontrast: Lumina of both aneurysm and pseudoaneurysm as well as their communication may be enhanced
CT Findings
- Additional CT findings
  - Anterior displacement of kidney by hematoma
  - Enlargement or obscuration of psoas muscle
  - Focally indistinct aortic margin that corresponds to site of rupture
  - Disruption of calcification of the aortic wall
MR Findings
- MRI has not been commonly used to evaluate patients suspected of having rupture of AAA

AAA with Rupture

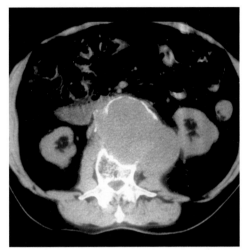

Nonenhanced CT scan. Contained rupture of aortic aneurysm. The mass is extending from the aorta into the psoas muscle, displacing the left kidney anteriorly. The process appears to be longstanding, note the erosion of the vertebral body.

- Findings will be similar to CT findings, although calcifications will not be evident

Ultrasound Findings
- Findings of AAA, may demonstrate intraperitoneal fluid
- Ultrasound is not accurate for determining presence of rupture

Imaging Recommendations
- Patients presenting with sudden onset of abdominal pain and a pulsatile abdominal mass should be taken directly to surgery without any further diagnostic tests
- CT is the imaging modality of choice for the evaluation of suspected rupture

Differential Diagnosis

Contained Rupture of the Aorta
- Rupture of the aorta which is contained in the retroperitoneum

Aortic Enteric Fistula
- Aortic aneurysm can rupture into the GI tract causing massive GI bleeding
- Clinically may present with hypovolemia, abdominal pain, and a pulsatile mass

Aortocaval Fistula
- Aortic aneurysm can rupture into the inferior vena cava
- May present with cardiac decompensation, and a pulsatile mass in the abdomen

Pathology

General
- General Path Comments
  o Location

AAA with Rupture

- • Rupture usually occurs into the left retroperitoneal space
- Etiology-Pathogenesis
  - o Risk of rupture is related to the size of the aneurysm
  - o Other risk factors for rupture
    - • Hypertension, chronic obstructive pulmonary disease (COPD), bronchiectasis, smoking, family history of AAA
- Epidemiology
  - o Approximate rates of rupture per year are
    - • If less than 4 cm in diameter, 0%
    - • If 4-5 cm in diameter, 0.5-5%
    - • If 5-6 cm in diameter, 10-20%
    - • If greater than 8 cm in diameter, 30-50%

Clinical Issues
Presentation
- Abrupt onset of severe central abdominal or back pain, occasionally localized to the lower abdomen, groin, or testes
- Pulsatile, usually tender abdominal mass
  - o AAA may be palpable in 50%
  - o May be absent due to hypotension
- Shock
  - o Some patients with a small, contained rupture may have a stable blood pressure

Treatment
- Surgical repair must be performed as soon as the diagnosis is made
- Rapid and maintained replacement of blood loss with crystalloid and blood transfusion to correct hypotension
- At this time in most cases percutaneous repair not appropriate

Prognosis
- Operative mortality rates range from 50-75%
- Death is usually secondary to massive intraoperative hemorrhage and cardiac complications

Selected References
1. Hartnell GG: Imaging of aortic aneurysms and dissection: CT and MRI. J Thorac Imaging 16: 35-46, 2001
2. Hallett JW: Management of abdominal aortic aneurysms. Mayo Clin Proc 75: 395-9, 2000
3. Yeung BK et al: Surgical management of abdominal aortic aneurysm. Vasc Med 5: 187-93, 2000

Celiac / SMA Occlusive Disease

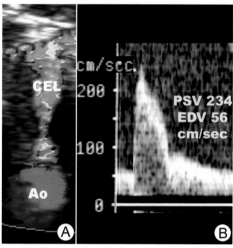

Celiac stenosis. (A) Color Doppler image shows narrowing of the celiac (CEL) origin and considerable post-stenotic flow disturbance (Ao=aorta). (B) Peak systolic velocity (PSV) and end diastolic velocity (EDV), respectively, 234 cm/sec and 56 cm/sec.

Key Facts
- Synonym: Mesenteric occlusive disease
- Definition: Stenosis or occlusion of the celiac artery and/or superior mesenteric artery (SMA), possibly causing mesenteric ischemia
- Classic imaging appearance
  - Narrowing or occlusion of the celiac artery or SMA
  - Flow reversal in the common hepatic artery with celiac occlusion
  - Mesenteric collateralization with SMA occlusion
- Other key facts
  - May contribute to acute mesenteric ischemia
  - Chronic mesenteric ischemia generally requires stenosis/occlusion of 2 out of 3 mesenteric arteries (celiac, SMA, inferior mesenteric artery (IMA))

Imaging Findings
General Features
- Best imaging clue
  - Stenosis/occlusion of celiac or SMA
  - Collateral flow

CTA and MRA Findings
- Celiac or SMA stenosis
- Celiac or SMA occlusion
- Possible post-stenotic dilation
- Celiac collateralization
  - Gastroduodenal artery to common hepatic artery, then to liver and spleen
  - Pancreatic bed collaterals to splenic artery
- SMA collateralization
  - Gastroduodenal artery to inferior pancreaticoduodenal arcade to small branches

Celiac / SMA Occlusive Disease

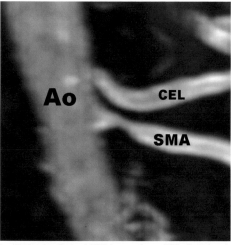

SMA stenosis. Contrast-enhanced MRA image shows 50% diameter stenosis of the SMA origin. The celiac artery (CEL) is widely patent. It is unlikely that this SMA stenosis would cause mesenteric ischemia.

- o IMA branches to SMA branches
- o Mesenteric collaterals (arch of Riolan, marginal artery of Drummond)
- Gadolinium enhancement required for MRA

Ultrasound Findings
- Color Doppler
  - o Occlusion or visible celiac/SMA narrowing, post-stenotic turbulence
  - o Flow reversal, gastroduodenal and common hepatic arteries
- Spectral Doppler
  - o Low resistance SMA Doppler waveforms in fasting patient (normally high resistance fasting, low resistance post-prandial)
  - o Doppler criteria, clinically significant stenosis (= 70% diameter)
    - Celiac = 200 cm/sec peak systole, 55 cm/sec end diastole
    - SMA = 275 cm/sec peak systole, 45 cm/sec end diastole

Other Modality Findings
- DSA, same as CTA/MRA

Imaging Recommendations
- Chronic mesenteric ischemia: CTA, MRA, and ultrasound all highly accurate, 85-95% sensitive/specific
- Acute mesenteric ischemia, use contrast-enhanced CT

Differential Diagnosis
Median Arcuate Ligament Compression of Celiac Origin
- Compression, during expiration, of celiac artery by the median arcuate ligament of the diaphragm
- Celiac stenosis on CTA, MRA or ultrasound **in expiration, relieved with deep inspiration**
- Dubious clinical symptoms (median arcuate ligament syndrome)

Celiac / SMA Occlusive Disease

Pathology

<u>General</u>
- Etiology-Pathogenesis
  - o Usual cause is atherosclerosis
  - o Fibromuscular dysplasia, arteritis, additional causes
- Anatomy
  - o Median acuate ligament
- Epidemiology
  - o Mesentric ischemia is generally a disease of the elderly
  - o Usually with risk factors for, and evidence of atherosclerosis

Clinical Issues

<u>Presentation</u>
- Celiac/SMA occlusive disease often is asymptomatic
- Chronic mesenteric ischemia
  - o Symptoms: Post-prandial pain and weight loss (frequently misinterpreted as cancer symptoms)
  - o Usually 2 of 3 major splanchnic arteries (celiac, SMA, IMA) stenotic/occluded when symptomatic
  - o Occasionally symptoms can occur with single vessel involvement
- Acute mesenteric ischemia
  - o Abdominal pain
  - o Usually due to embolus to SMA
  - o Distention
  - o Ileus
  - o Possible peritoneal signs
  - o Elevated serum lactate

<u>Natural History</u>
- Progressive, with advancement of atherosclerosis

<u>Treatment</u>
- Angioplasty/stent
- Surgical bypass

<u>Prognosis</u>
- If single vessel, may remain asymptomatic
- Chronic mesenteric ischemia: Progressive weight loss, disability

Selected References
1. Zwolak RM: Can duplex ultrasound replace arteriography in screening for mesenteric ischemia? Semin Vasc Surg 12(4): 252-60, 1999
2. Thomas JH et al: The clinical course of asymptomatic mesenteric arterial stenosis. J Vasc Surg 27: 840-4, 1998
3. Moneta GL et al: Mesenteric duplex scanning. A blinded prospective study. J Vasc Surg 17: 79-86, 1993

Portal Hypertension

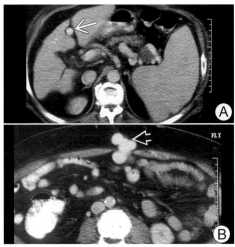

Portal hypertension (contrast-enhanced CT). (A) A large umbilical vein porto-systemic collateral (arrow) is seen in the ligamentum teres. The spleen is enlarged. (B) The umbilical vein collateral drains into large varices (open arrow) at the umbilicus.

Key Facts
- Definition: Elevated pressure in the portal venous system
- Classic imaging appearance
  - Dilatation of the portal vein (PV), splenic and mesenteric veins
  - Porto-systemic collaterals
  - Splenomegaly
- Other key facts
  - Hepatic vein wedge pressure 10 mm above IVC pressure
  - Most commonly caused by hepatic cirrhosis
  - Etiology may be pre-sinusoidal (PV occlusion), sinusoidal (usually cirrhosis) or post-sinusoidal (hepatic vein/IVC obstruction)
  - Presents with upper GI hemorrhage from collaterals

Imaging Findings
Best Imaging Clues
- Dilated PV, portosystemic collaterals

CT/MR Findings
- Dilated PV (> 17 mm with deep inspiration)
- Portosystemic collaterals
  - Gastroesophageal (coronary vein/left gastric, right gastric/ splenogastric)
  - Splenorenal
  - Recanalized umbilical vein
  - Mesenteric/retroperitoneal
- Hepatic cirrhosis
  - Surface nodularity, small right lobe, enlarged left/caudate lobes
  - Note: If cirrhotic changes are present, PH is present
- Splenomegaly
- Ascites
- Possible PV thrombosis

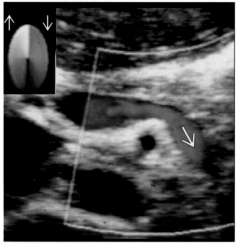

Reversed splenic vein flow in portal hypertension. The color wheel (upper left) indicates that flow away from the transducer is colored blue. Thus, splenic vein flow is away from the portal vein (PV) and toward the spleen, which is the reverse of normal (arrow).

- Cavernous transformation of thrombosed PV
  - Tangle of collateral veins in porta hepatis/peripancreatic area
  - Absent PV, possibly splenic vein as well

<u>Ultrasound Findings</u>
- Same as above, plus
- PV > 13 mm in quiet respiration, supine subject
- Less than 20% increase in splenic vein/SMV diameter from quiet respiration to deep inspiration (normally increase 50-100%)
- Possible flow reversal in PV or splenic vein (definitive finding)

<u>Catheter Angiography</u>
- Wedge hepatic vein (portal sinusoid) pressure 10 mmHg > IVC

<u>Imaging Recommendations</u>
- Ultrasound for primary diagnosis of portal hypertension (PH)/PV occlusion
- CT/MRI if US technically impaired, and pre-transplantation
- Advanced methods for portal flow measurement
- DSA for therapy (see below)

Differential Diagnosis
<u>Splenic Vein Occlusion</u>
- Mimics portal hypertension findings
  - Large spleno-renal, spleno-gastric, gastroesophageal collateral veins
  - Splenomegaly
  - Gastroesophageal hemorrhage
- Always think of this diagnosis with large splenic collaterals
- Confirm/exclude by looking for splenic vein

<u>Congestive Heart Failure</u>
- Distended hepatic veins, PVs, IVC
- Hepatomegaly
- Ascites

Portal Hypertension

Pathology

<u>General</u>
- PH may result from PV obstruction (pre-sinusoidal), hepatocellular disease (sinusoidal) or hepatic vein/IVC obstruction (post-sinusoidal)
- Anatomy
  - All gut and spleen blood flow normally passes through the liver
  - Portal venous system unique: Veins connecting two capillary systems
- Epidemiology
  - Chronic active hepatitis and schistosomiasis are major cause of PH morbidity and mortality

<u>Etiology-Pathogenesis</u>
- Pre-sinusoidal
  - PV occlusion unrelated to liver disease
    - Acute pancreatitis
    - Septic PV phlebitis (e.g., appendiceal abscess, Crohn's disease)
    - Severe dehydration, especially in children
    - Hypercoagulable states (primary or malignancy related)
  - Tumor growth into PV (usually hepatocellular carcinoma)
  - Schistosomiasis: Parasitic periportal fibrosis
  - Congenital hepatic fibrosis (infancy, childhood)
  - Primary biliary cirrhosis (adulthood)
  - Sarcoidosis
- Sinusoidal obstruction
  - Cirrhosis: Lobular scarring and regeneration due to toxins (especially alcohol) and chronic active hepatitis (B & C)
- PH in advanced cirrhosis complicated by increased splanchnic arterial flow
- Post sinusoidal
- See "Budd-Chiari Syndrome"

Clinical Issues

<u>Presentation</u>
- Acute GI hemorrhage (variceal)
- Hepatic dysfunction, liver failure
- Ascites
- PH often an **important incidental finding** on imaging studies
  - Risk of hemorrhage at surgery
  - Risk of spontaneous variceal hemorrhage

<u>Natural History</u>
- Progressive when due to cirrhosis

<u>Treatment</u>
- Endoscopic sclerotherapy for gastroesophageal hemorrhage
- Transjugular intrahepatic portocaval shunt (TIPS)
- Surgical portosystemic shunt

<u>Prognosis</u>
- Guarded due to progression of liver disease and/or shunt failure

Selected References
1. Vosshenrich R et al: Contrast-enhanced MR angiography of abdominal vessels. Eur Radiol 12: 218-301, 2002
2. Martínez-Noguera A et al: Doppler in hepatic cirrhosis and chronic hepatitis. Semin Ultrasound CT MR 23: 19-36, 2002
3. Pieters PC et al: Evaluation of the portal venous system: complementary roles of invasive and noninvasive imaging strategies. Radiographics 17: 879-952, 1997

Budd-Chiari Syndrome

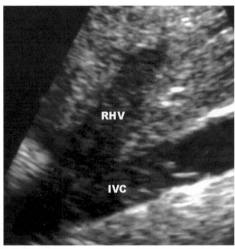

Acute Budd-Chiari syndrome. A coronal US image shows occlusive material in the right hepatic vein (RHV) and the IVC, subsequently proven to be hepatocellular carcinoma.

Key Facts
- Definition: Budd-Chiari Syndrome = acute onset of abdominal pain, hepatic dysfunction, ascites, and (possible) lower extremity swelling, caused by obstruction of the IVC and/or hepatic veins (HVs)
- Classic imaging appearance
  - Obstructed HVs and/or IVC
  - Portal venous congestion
  - Intrahepatic collaterals
  - "Spider web" pattern of hepatic veins (hepatic venography)
- Other key facts
  - Obstruction of at least two HVs for Budd-Chiari syndrome
  - Neoplastic or thrombotic etiology

Imaging Findings
General Features
- Best imaging clue: IVC and/or HV occlusion
- Contrast enhancement required for CT
- Time-of-flight or contrast-enhanced images for MRI
CTA and MRA Findings
- Acute
  - Visible occlusion, or severe stenosis, of at least two HVs and/or IVC
  - Hepatomegaly
  - Edema, decreased enhancement in segments with obstructed HVs
  - Portal/splanchnic veins distended (portal hypertension)
  - Ascites
  - Portosystemic collaterals (intrahepatic and/or extrahepatic)
  - HV-to-HV collaterals (intrahepatic)
  - Possible tumor enhancement IVC/HVs
  - Possible neoplastic mass (intrahepatic or extrahepatic)
  - Low signal T1, high signal T2 in liver periphery

Budd-Chiari Syndrome

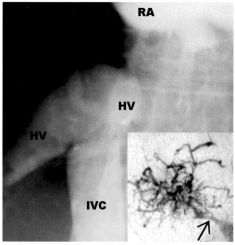

Contrast venogram, and simultaneous right atrial (RA) injection, showing IVC occlusion (neoplastic). Although HVs were open, patient presented with the Budd-Chiari syndrome. Hepatic venogram (insert: different patient) showing the spider web pattern of intrahepatic collaterals and a stenosed, recanalized HV (arrow).

- Chronic
  - Loss of volume/scar of hepatic segments subtended by obstructed HVs, (interlobar distribution)
  - Possible recanalization of HVs/IVC (stenotic/irregular lumen)
  - Portal hypertension
  - Portosystemic collaterals (intrahepatic and/or extrahepatic)
  - HV-to-HV collaterals (intrahepatic)
  - Possible ascites
  - IVC/iliac vein congestion and collaterals (with IVC obstruction)

<u>Ultrasound Findings</u>
- Same as CT/MRI, plus
  - Possible flow reversal in portal vein branches and IVC
  - Continuous flow pattern in portal vein, and/or in IVC/extremity veins (no respiratory variation)
  - Possible tumor vascularity in HV and IVC (tumor thrombus)

<u>DSA Findings</u>
- Occluded, stenotic or recanalized HVs and IVC on venography
- Classic **spider web pattern** of intrahepatic HV branches
- Intrahepatic portosystemic or HV-to-HV collaterals

<u>Imaging Recommendations</u>
- Ultrasound for confirming/excluding Budd-Chiari syndrome
- MRA or CTA when US technically limited
- MRA or CTA for definitive diagnosis and etiology
- DSA for vascular diagnosis, treatment

Differential Diagnosis
<u>Acute or Chronic Hepatic Failure</u>
- Cirrhosis
- Acute hepatitis

Budd-Chiari Syndrome

Right Heart Failure
- IVC/HV congestion mimics clinical Budd-Chiari syndrome

Pathology
General
- Three potential causes of Budd-Chiari
  - o IVC obstruction
  - o HV obstruction
  - o Occlusion of HVs in hepatic sinusoids (uncommon)
    - Rare cause of Budd-Chiari
    - Potentially undetectable by CT/MRI/US if HVs remain patent
    - Classic findings on liver biopsy
- Anatomy
  - o Intrahepatic vascular connections exist normally (HV-to-HV and HVs-to-portal veins) but are rarely seen in healthy individuals
  - o Connections enlarge in Budd-Chiari (and in cirrhosis)
- Etiology-Pathogenesis
  - o Thrombosis of HVs
    - Stasis-reduced blood flow in cirrhosis/portal hypertension
    - Hypercoagulability (primary or neoplasm-induced)
    - Severe dehydration
  - o Malignant neoplasm
    - Hepatocellular carcinoma with HV/IVC invasion (most common)
    - Extrinsic HV/IVC compression or invasion
    - Rare vascular sarcoma
  - o Rare "congenital" obstruction of IVC

Clinical Issues
Presentation
- Variable: Depends on rapidity of obstructive process and collateralization
- Classical: Acute onset of abdominal pain, hepatomegaly and ascites, plus lower extremity edema with IVC obstruction
- Subacute/chronic: Hepatic failure, ascites, distended veins on abdomen, variceal bleeding, plus lower extremity edema with IVC obstruction
Treatment
- Anticoagulation with thrombotic occlusion
- Angioplasty of recanalized IVC, HVs
- TIPS if sufficient HV recanalization
- Surgical porto-systemic shunt
Prognosis
- Variable, depending on etiology, collateralization, HV recanalization
- Persistence of HV obstruction is likely, causing
  - o Hepatic failure/cirrhosis
  - o Variceal bleeding
  - o Intractable ascites
- Neoplastic obstruction usually is fatal

Selected References
1. Noone TC et al: Budd-Chiari syndrome: spectrum of appearances of acute, subacute, and chronic disease with magnetic resonance imaging. J Magn Reson Imaging 11: 44-501, 2000
2. Chawla Y et al: Duplex Doppler sonography in patients with Budd-Chiari syndrome. J Gastroenterol Hepatol 14: 904-7, 1999
3. Okuda H et al: Epidemiological and clinical features of Budd-Chiari syndrome in Japan. J Hepatol 22: 1-9, 1995

Portal Vein Occlusion

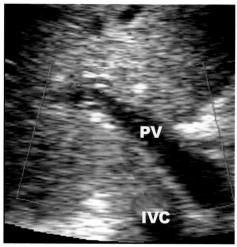

Acute portal vein thrombosis. The portal vein (PV) is filled with low-echogenicity thrombus. No flow is present, even though flow is detected readily in the IVC.

Key Facts
- Definition: Occlusion of the portal vein (PV) due to thrombosis or tumor invasion
- Classic imaging appearance
  - Absence of blood flow or filling defect in the PV
  - Cavernous transformation of the PV (collateralization in the porta hepatitis)
- Other key facts
  - Commonly associated with hepatic cirrhosis and pancreatitis
  - Presentation varies from acute symptoms to unrecognized clinically

Imaging Findings
<u>General Features</u>
- Best imaging clue
  - Visualized PV with absence of flow or flow void
  - Non-visualization of the PV (chronic occlusion)
  - Cavernous transformation
<u>CT Findings</u>
- Contrast is essential for accurate CT diagnosis
- Acute PV thrombosis
  - Non-occlusive: Low-density thrombus partially filling **patent** PV
  - Occlusive: Low-density thrombus filling **dilated** portal vein
    - Extent variable: May include major intrahepatic branches, splenic vein and superior mesenteric vein (SMV)
    - Congested (non-occluded) mesenteric veins distal to thrombus
    - Possible bowel wall edema
    - Possible ileus
    - Possible ascites
    - Possible splenomegaly
- Chronic PV thrombosis

Portal Vein Occlusion

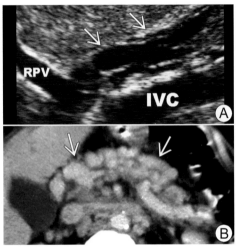

Cavernous transformation & collateralization. (A) US image showing cavernous transformation (arrows) of PV (RPV=right portal vein). (B) CT in the same patient shows massive collateralization (arrows) in pancreatic bed. Also note collaterals adjacent to aorta. Patient was asymptomatic! Probable cause, pancreatitis.

- o Non-visualization of PV, possibly also splenic vein (thrombosed vein becomes fibrotic "cord" not visible on imaging studies)
- o Cavernous transformation of PV: Large collaterals along the usual course of PV, possibly with peripancreatic, splenic vein collaterals
- o Well-developed portosystemic collaterals, as in portal hypertension
- o Possible splenomegaly
- o Possible atrophy/nodular regeneration of ischemic liver segments
- o Possible increased hepatic artery size and flow
- PV tumor invasion
  - o Similar to acute thrombosis, but
  - o Variable degree of contrast enhancement of intraluminal tumor
  - o Primary tumor usually visible in hepatic parenchyma, or pancreas

MR Findings
- Analogous to CT findings
- Acute thrombus-low signal flow void in PV
- Subacute thrombus-hyperintense on T1 and T2 due to methemoglobin
- Contrast enhanced MRA more accurate than TOF and phase contrast
- Liver parenchyma supplied by thrombosed veins may enhance avidly in arterial phase; due to increased hepatic artery flow
- PV tumor enhances avidly, especially on GRE sequences

Ultrasound (US) Findings
- Analogous to CT
- Tumor vessels usually visible in intraluminal tumor on color Doppler

Imaging Recommendations
- US initially: Highly accurate and cost effective
- Contrast CT for comprehensive evaluation/search for cause
- MRI as alternative for CT
- Direct splenoportogram gives excellent visualization

Portal Vein Occlusion

Differential Diagnosis
Sluggish PV Flow Due to Cirrhosis
- May mimic occlusion on Doppler US and non-contrast MRA
- No cavernous transformation

Splenic Vein Occlusion
- Massive splenic-systemic collateral network mimics PV occlusion
- Patent PV, absence of splenic vein

Pathology
General
- PV occlusion is uncommon
- Most frequently seen in cirrhotic patients
- Anatomy
  - Venous flow from bowel/spleen normally traverses PV
  - PV occlusion = extensive portosystemic collateral network
  - Increased size and flow hepatic artery due to decreased PV flow
- Etiology-Pathogenesis
  - Thrombosis
    - Stasis from cirrhosis-related sinusoidal obstruction
    - Acute pancreatitis
    - Seeding of PV by infected material (acute appendicitis, intraperitoneal abscess, inflammatory bowel disease)
    - Hypercoagulable states (primary or tumor-related)
  - Tumor invasion
    - Hepatocellular carcinoma most common
    - Pancreatic carcinoma
    - Liver metastases

Clinical Issues
Presentation
- Liver dysfunction
- Abdominal pain (from bowel congestion, ileus, rare venous infarction)
- Possible ascites
- Incidental finding on imaging study (see image on previous page)
  - Common incidental finding in advanced cirrhosis
  - Also seen in healthy, non-cirrhotic individual with unrecognized, previous PV thrombosis (e.g., from acute pancreatitis, now resolved)

Prognosis
- Non-occlusive PV thrombosis may lyse = no residua or minor PV scarring
- Occlusive PV thrombosis = permanent PV occlusion
  - Portal hypertension morbidity (gastrointestinal hemorrhage)
  - Reduced hepatic blood flow, possible tissue death, regeneration
- PV tumor invasion is fatal

Treatment
- Supportive therapy only
- Anticoagulation for acute thrombosis (if liver function permits)

Selected References
1. Bradbury MS et al: Noninvasive assessment of portomesenteric venous thrombosis: current concepts and imaging strategies. J Comput Assist Tomogr 26(3): 392-404, 2002
2. Kreft B et al: Detection of thrombosis in the portal venous system: comparison of contrast-enhanced MRA with intraarterial DSA. Radiology 216: 86-92, 2000
3. Bach AM et al: Portal vein evaluation with US: comparison to angiography combined with CT arterial portography. Radiology 201(1): 149-154, 1996

TIPS Follow-Up

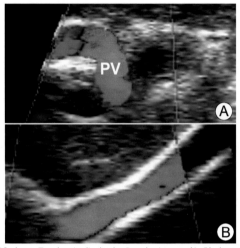

Normal TIPS shunt. Two longitudinal color Doppler images (A, B) show the brightly echogenic walls of the TIPS stent. Note that color (flow) extends to the wall, and that the stent ends are well positioned within the hepatic and portal veins (PV).

Key Facts
- Definition: TIPS = **T**ransjugular **I**ntrahepatic **P**ortocaval **S**hunt
- Classic imaging appearance
  - Intrahepatic metallic stent connecting the hepatic venous system with the portal venous system
  - High flow velocity in portal vein (PV)
- Stent usually extends from right hepatic vein (HV) to right PV, near confluence with main PV
- Stent placed as follows
  - Internal jugular vein (preferably right) cannulated percutaneously
  - Catheterization of HV
  - Penetration of liver by needle until the right PV is reached, wire then catheter placed into portal vein forming intrahepatic tract
  - Intrahepatic tract balloon dilatated
  - Placement of balloon-expandable metallic stent in intrahepatic tract

Imaging Findings
General Features
- Best imaging clue: Metallic stent, with blood flow, connecting HV and PV
- TIPS failure
  - Stent malposition or kink
  - Focal stenosis
    - Most often in draining HV, development of intimal hyperplasia
    - Neointimal hyperplasia in stent
  - Fusiform or diffuse stenosis from neointimal hyperplasia
- Susceptibility artifact from metal stent limits follow-up value of MRA
Pre-TIPS US Evaluation
- Confirm patency of
  - Internal jugular vein
  - HVs

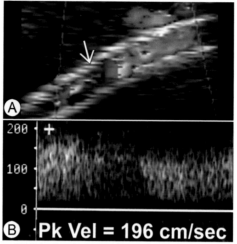

TIPS stenosis. (A) Color Doppler image shows considerable narrowing of the shunt (arrow). (B) Peak velocity in the narrowed area is very high (196 cm/sec). Peak velocity in the PV (not shown) was only 14 cm/sec (normally 35-45 cm/sec).

-     o PVs
- Confirm that right and left portal branches unite within liver (risk of hemorrhage with extrahepatic union)
- Document
  - Flow direction in right, left and main PVs, and splenic vein
  - Peak flow velocity in main PV

Post-TIPS CT Findings
- IV contrast enhancement, timing for portal phase essential (triple-phase liver technique)
- Satisfactory
  - Ends of stent squarely centered HV, PV
  - Straight stent or smooth curve, no kinks
  - Prompt contrast opacification of stent
  - Contrast extends to stent walls (no filling defect)
  - Fairly uniform vein/stent caliber (no focal narrowing)
  - Hepatopetal flow in main PV and splenic vein
- Unsatisfactory
  - Poor centering/kinking of stent
  - Absence of stent flow
  - Delayed stent opacification, compared with splenic vein/collaterals
  - Stenosis: Fusiform or focal, stent or HV
  - Hepatofugal flow in splenic vein

Post-TIPS Ultrasound Findings
- Satisfactory
  - As above for CT
  - Turbulence is normal in stent
  - Mild pulsatility is common
  - Stent velocity (peak)
    - Similar at portal and hepatic ends
    - Usually 90-120 cm/sec

- Minimal normal: 50-60 cm/sec
  - PV velocity (peak)
    - Usual range 35-45 cm/sec
    - Minimum 30 cm/sec
  - Hepatopetal PV, splenic vein flow (left PV may remain reversed)
- Unsatisfactory
  - Localized stenosis with high velocity/turbulence
  - > 100 cm/sec increase in velocity from one point to another in stent
  - Diffuse narrowing, with or without high velocity
  - Generalized low velocity
  - Decreased PV velocity from post-procedure baseline
  - PV velocity < 30 cm/sec
  - Hepatofugal or biphasic PV or splenic vein flow
  - Absence of flow in shunt (**always confirm occlusion with DSA**)

Imaging Recommendations
- US for primary pre/post TIPS assessment
- CT when US technically compromised
- DSA to confirm occlusion or treat stenosis (angioplasty)

Differential Diagnosis
Surgical Porto-Systemic Shunt
- Extrahepatic location
Spontaneous Intrahepatic Porto-Hepatic Shunt
- No stent

Pathology
- None

Clinical Issues
Natural History
- Hepatic diseases leading to TIPS shunting are progressive
Indications for TIPS
- Palliative procedure for intractable ascites, recurrent gastrointestinal hemorrhage
- Temporizing measure while awaiting liver transplantation
- Surgical shunts may be more appropriate in selected patients
Prognosis
- High stenosis/occlusion rate
  - 66% one-year patency without intervention
  - 88% one-year patency with intervention
- No effect on underlying liver disease/liver failure
- Patients with severe liver disease may develop liver failure, TIPS following

Selected References
1. Chopra S: Transjugular intrahepatic portosystemic shunt: Accuracy of helical CT angiography in the detection of shunt abnormalities. Radiology 215: 115-22, 2000
2. Zwiebel WJ: Vascular disorders of the liver. in Zwiebel WJ ed: Introduction to Vascular Ultrasonography (Ed 4), Philadelphia, W.B. Saunders, 431-54, 2000
3. Tesdal IK: Transjugular intrahepatic portosystemic shunting (TIPS) with balloon-expandable and self-expanding stents: Technical and clinical aspects after 3-1/2 years' experience. Cardiovasc Intervent Radiol 20: 29-37, 1997

PocketRadiologist™
Vascular
Top 100 Diagnoses

RENAL

Polyarteritis Nodosa

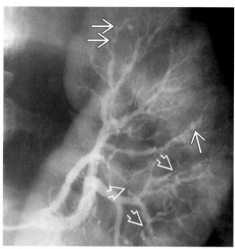

Polyarteritis nodosa of the renal arterial vasculature. Multiple small aneurysms in many branches of the renal arteries (arrows). Also multiple focal areas of stenoses (open arrows). Numerous regions of ectasia present throughout renal arteries.

Key Facts
- Synonym: PAN, Kussmaul-Maier disease
- Definition: A systemic inflammatory vasculitis, characterized by necrotizing inflammatory foci in walls of small and medium sized arteries
- Classic imaging appearance: Multiple, small, aneurysms on angiography
- Overlap with imaging findings seen in other necrotizing vasculitis (SLE, Wegener's granulomatosis, rheumatoid vasculitis, drug abuse)

Imaging Findings
General Features
- Best imaging clue: Multiple, 1-5 mm peripheral aneurysms in vessels of the kidney, mesentery, and liver
  - Occlusions
  - Irregular stenoses throughout the abdominal viscera vessels
CT Findings
- Demonstrate large aneurysms, stenosis and occlusions of larger vessels
- Demonstrate organ involvement, with regions of ischemia/infarction
- Exclude malignancy, or trauma as causes for aneurysms
MR Findings
- Demonstrate large aneurysms, stenosis and occlusions of larger vessels
- Demonstrate organ involvement, with regions of ischemia/infarction
- Exclude malignancy, or trauma as causes for aneurysms
Angiography
- Multiple small-sized aneurysms, ectasia, stenoses, and occlusions
Imaging Recommendations
- Angiographic detection of multiple small-sized aneurysms is necessary to specifically diagnose PAN
- CTA and MRA can detect abnormalities in more advanced disease
- CT provides good visualization of organ changes and complications

Polyarteritis Nodosa

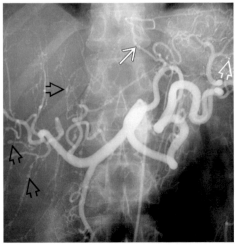

Polyarteritis nodosa involving multiple arteries. Liver with numerous small aneurysms (black open arrows). Spleen with aneurysms (white open arrow). Gastric artery with ectasia (white arrow). (Courtesy John Kaufman, MD)

Differential Diagnosis
Microscopic Polyangiitis
- Small-sized vessels affected
- Usually characterized by presence of glomerulonephritis and pulmonary involvement

Systemic Lupus Erythematosus (SLE)
- Causes both arterial and venous thrombotic vascular changes
- Raynaud's phenomenon present in up to 30% of patients
- Angiographically, small and medium sized vessels show tapered or abrupt occlusions with sparse formation of collateral vessels

Pathology
General
- General Path Comments
  - Can involve any organ and in varying degrees
  - Kidneys involved in 70-80% of cases
  - GI tract, peripheral nerves, skin in 50%
  - Skeletal muscles, mesentery in 30%
  - CNS in 10%
  - Heart, testicles, lung, and spleen rarely involved
- Etiology-Pathogenesis
  - Thought to be a result of immune-complex deposition
  - Possible causative agents
  - Hepatitis B, HIV
  - Other viruses
  - Hematological disease (hairy-cell leukemia)
- Epidemiology
  - Annual incidence: 0.7 per 100,000
  - Annual prevalence: 6.3 per 100,000
  - Predominant sex: Female > Male (2:1)

- o Predominant age of onset: 40-60 years

Microscopic Features

- Acute phase of arterial wall inflammation
  - o Fibrinoid necrosis of the media, destruction of elastic lamina
  - o Intense pleomorphic cellular infiltration
  - o Normal architecture completely effaced and replaced by a band of amorphous eosinophilic material
- Arterial healing characterized by fibrotic endarteritis

Staging or Grading Criteria

- Five factor score (FFS)
  - o Proteinuria > 1g/day
  - o Renal insufficiency (creatinine > 140 mg/DL)
  - o Cardiomyopathy
  - o GI symptoms
  - o CNS involvement

Clinical Issues

Presentation

- Varied spectrum of organ involvement, wide range of clinical symptoms, and variation in severity
  - o Abdominal pain
  - o Hypertension
  - o Arthralgia/arthritis
  - o PNS and CNS dysfunction
  - o Cardiac, respiratory, hepatic involvement

Natural History

- Untreated, 5-year survival < 15%

Treatment

- Medical treatment
- Glucocorticoids as first line treatment
- Cyclophosphamide, depending on severity/intensity of disease activity
- Azathioprine for patients with contraindications to cyclophosphamide
- Plasma exchanges in PAN refractory to conventional therapy
- Surgery may be need to treat bowel perforation

Prognosis

- FFS prognostic
  - o FFS=0, mortality at 5 years 12%
  - o FFS=1, mortality at 5 years 26%
  - o FFS > 2, mortality at 5 years 46%
- Glucocorticoid treatment increase 5-year survival from 15-80%
- Low relapse rate

Selected References
1. Guillevin L: Polyarteritis nodosa and microscopic polyangiitis. In: Ball GV and Bridges SL, ed. Vasculitis. 1st ed.: 300-21, 2002
2. Stanson AS: Polyarteritis nodosa: Spectrum of angiographic findings. Radiographics 21: 151-9, 2001
3. Gee KN: Radiologic findings of abdominal polyarteritis nodosa. AJR 174: 1675-9, 2000

Renal Artery Stenosis

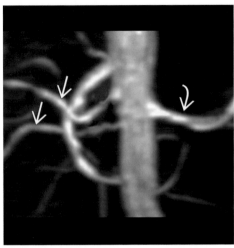

Gadolinium-enhanced, reformatted MRA shows a lengthy stenosis of about 50% diameter reduction in the left renal artery (curved arrow). Duplicate main renal arteries are present on the right (arrows), with a high-grade stenosis in the superior artery.

Key Facts
- Definition: Narrowing of a renal artery (RA), possibly leading to renal ischemia
- Classic imaging appearance
  - CTA, MRA, DSA: RA narrowing, possibly with post-stenotic dilatation
  - Ultrasound (US): RA narrowing with high velocity flow/turbulence
- Other key facts
  - Therapeutic benefit of stenosis repair remains controversial

Imaging Findings
CTA/MRA/DSA Findings
- Contrast enhancement and multiplanar reformat required for CTA/DSA
- Focal or multifocal narrowing of one or more renal artery
- Post-stenotic dilatation (suggests hemodynamic significance)
- Web-like lesions, beaded appearance with fibromuscular dysplasia
- Classify stenosis as > 50% or > 70% diameter reduction
- Be conscious of duplicate main RAs and accessory RAs

US Findings
- Focal RA narrowing on color Doppler images
- High velocity in the narrowed area
  - Peak systolic velocity 280-300 cm/sec or greater
  - RA / aortic ratio $\geq$ 3.5 (peak systole RA stenosis/peak systole aorta at level of RAs)
- Post stenotic disturbed flow
- Possible damped Doppler waveforms and delayed systolic acceleration (< 0.07 sec) distal to stenosis in RA, or in segmental/lobar branches
  - Seen only with > 70% diameter narrowing
  - May be obscured by high resistance from renal parenchymal disease

Imaging Recommendations
- CTA/MRA vs. US

Renal Artery Stenosis

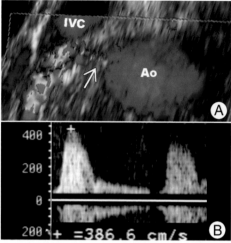

Renal artery stenosis. (A) Color Doppler image shows a tight stenosis (arrow) of the right renal artery (Ao=aorta). (B) Doppler spectrum analysis: Peak systolic velocity 386 cm/sec, renal/aorta ratio (not shown on image) 7.0. Both measures indicate a high-grade stenosis exceeding 70% diameter reduction.

- o Some institutions recommend US, which is less costly than CTA/MRA
  - ▪ US best for atherosclerotic lesions (RA origin)
  - ▪ US ineffective for distal/hilar stenoses (fibromuscular dysplasia)
  - ▪ US often misses duplicate/accessory renal arteries
  - ▪ Frequent technical difficulties due to bowel contents, obesity
- o CTA and MRA preferred by other institutions
  - ▪ High success rate and greater accuracy than US in some series
  - ▪ Duplicate/accessory arteries visualized
  - ▪ Hilar stenoses not seen with MRA
- o DSA for indeterminate CT/MRI and for therapy

Differential Diagnosis
Renal Artery Occlusion
- Non-visualization of RA with US, CT, MRI
- Small kidney size (8 cm or less)
- Blood supply from capsular collaterals

Pathology
General
- General Path Comments
  - o Significant RA stenosis causes renal ischemia and release of renin, which is converted to angiotensin, ultimately causing systemic hypertension
- Embryology-Anatomy
  - o Duplicate RAs present in up to 30% of kidneys
  - o Duplicate main RAs
    - ▪ Large size, arise from aorta, supply hilar branches
    - ▪ Stenosis may cause hypertension
  - o Polar accessory arteries

Renal Artery Stenosis

- Small size, aorta or iliac artery to lower pole
- Stenosis causing hypertension, depends on amount of kidney affected
- Etiology-Pathogenesis
  - Atherosclerosis
    - Most common cause of stenosis/occlusion, usually at RA origin
    - Elderly population
  - Fibromuscular dysplasia
    - Distal RA or hilar branches, may be multifocal
    - Young adults
  - Congenital stenosis (childhood)

Staging or Grading Criteria
- 50% diameter stenosis is hemodynamically significant
- High-grade stenosis ($\geq$ 70%) more likely to cause hypertension/ischemia

Clinical Issues

Epidemiology
- 5-10% of hypertension is caused by RA disease (less in some estimates)

Presentation
- Hypertension and/or renal failure
- When is imaging search for RA stenosis warranted?
  - Hypertension in childhood and young adults
  - Adult hypertension, uncontrolled with three or more drugs
  - Previously controlled hypertension now uncontrollable
  - Rapidly worsening (malignant) hypertension
  - Hypertension with deteriorating renal function

Treatment
- Indications for RA stenosis treatment remain controversial
  - Patient selection very important
  - Therapy for hypertension more widely accepted than for renal failure
- Balloon angioplasty/stent (most common)
  - Significant restenosis rate (about 20-25%)
  - Less risky than surgery
- Surgical bypass graft for selected indications
  - Durable results, low restenosis/occlusion rate

Prognosis
- Therapeutic benefit, hypertension (short term, well-selected adults)
  - Angioplasty/stent: About 70% cure or improved control
  - Surgical bypass: About 90% cure or improved control
- Therapeutic benefit, ischemic nephropathy
  - Disappointing results in relatively small series
  - Questionable indication for therapy

Selected References
1. Kimberly J et al: Renovascular Disease [in] Moore WS: Vascular surgery: A comprehensive review, ed 6. Philadelphia, WB Saunders, 548-69, 2002
2. Dawson DL: Noninvasive assessment of renal artery stenosis. Semin in Vasc Surg 9(3): 172-81, 1996
3. Miralles M et al: Value of Doppler parameters in the diagnosis of renal artery stenosis. J Vasc Surg 23: 428-35, 1996

Renal Vein Thrombosis

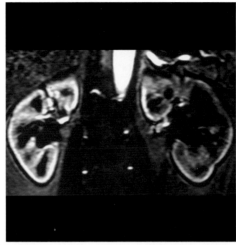

Acute RV thrombosis, arterial phase Gd enhanced 3D MRA. The left kidney is enlarged and hypoperfused overall (except the rim of cortex). A large non-perfused region is evident.

Key Facts
- Definition: Thrombus formation in the renal vein (RV), usually causing venous occlusion
- Classic imaging appearance
  - RV distended by non-enhancing thrombus
  - Absent blood flow
  - Striking alteration of renal parenchyma in acute thrombosis

Imaging Findings
General Features
- Best imaging clue: See classic imaging appearance
- Acute thrombosis findings well described, little information on chronic thrombosis
- MRA seems more accurate than CTA (multidetector CT not yet reported)
Findings (Acute Thrombosis)
- RV usually distended, thrombus may extend into inferior vena cava (IVC)
- RV thrombus: Hypodense CT, low signal T1 and T2 weighted MR images
- Possible "tram-track" of blood flow around thrombus on CTA and MRA
- Kidney is enlarged, massive in some cases
- Edema in perinephric and peripelvic fat (CT or MR)
- Parenchymal appearance, non-contrast CT
  - Diffusely hypodense
  - Possible areas of increased density from parenchymal hemorrhage
- Parenchymal appearance, contrast-enhanced CT
  - Diminished, but prolonged enhancement, due to congestion and failure of contrast to "wash out"
  - Prolonged conspicuity of corticomedullary contrast difference
  - Enhancement may be striated or heterogeneous, with focal non-enhancing areas, due to hemorrhagic necrosis
- Parenchymal appearance, non-enhanced MR

Renal Vein Thrombosis

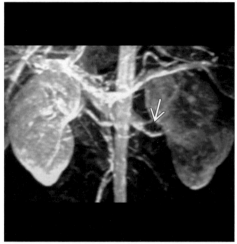

Venous phase MR image, in the same patient as previous page, shows thrombus (arrow) within the proximal left renal vein.

- o Overall diminished T1 and T2 signal
- o Absence of normally-seen corticomedullary signal differences
- o Possible areas with increased T1 **and** T2 signal, due to hemorrhage
- Parenchymal appearance, contrast-enhanced MR
  - o Diminished enhancement overall, due to congestion
  - o Enhancement may be heterogeneous, due to hemorrhagic necrosis
  - o Absent medullary enhancement (severe ischemia, infarction)

Findings (Subacute Thrombosis)
- Variable distention of RV
- Possible high signal in RV thrombus on T1 **and** T2 weighted MR images (methemoglobin)
- Numerous collateral veins around kidney, renal pelvis and proximal ureter (contrast CT, MR)

Findings (Chronic Thrombosis)
- Lysis of thrombus
  - o Recanalization of RV
  - o Return to normal parenchymal appearance (CT, MR, US)
- Persistent RV thrombosis (usual)
  - o RV occluded but not distended
  - o Numerous collateral veins around kidney, renal pelvis and proximal ureter (contrast CT, MR)
  - o Parenchyma may return to normal CT/MR appearance if collateralization is excellent (not necessarily normal function)
  - o Parenchyma may undergo progressive fibrosis, with decreased kidney size and homogeneous fibrotic appearance (loss of renal function)

Ultrasound (US) Findings (Acute Thrombosis)
- RV thrombus, low echogenicity, with absence of flow on color Doppler
- Enlarged kidney: Three possible parenchymal patterns
  - o Diffuse hypoechoic parenchyma, no corticomedullary difference
  - o Increased cortical echogenicity, retained corticomedullary difference
  - o Diffuse heterogeneity (from extensive hemorrhagic necrosis)

Renal Vein Thrombosis

- Linear, echogenic streaks radiating from hilus-said to be pathognomonic, attributed to acutely thrombosed parenchymal veins

Imaging Recommendations
- Color Doppler US, best modality in infants and small children
- MRA appears more accurate than CTA or US for direct visualization of RV thrombus (even without contrast), procedure of choice in adults
- CTA disadvantage: Nephrotoxic effects of contrast
- All modalities detect parenchymal abnormalities

Differential Diagnosis
RV Tumor Extension
- Tumor vascularity on US, tumor enhancement on contrast CT and MR

Acute Pyelonephritis
- RV patent

Diffuse Neoplastic Infiltration
- Lymphoma, leukemia, transitional cell- or renal cell carcinoma
- RV usually patent, possible RV tumor extension

Pathology
General
- General Path Comments
  - Nephrotic syndrome frequent cause of RV thrombosis, especially when due to membranous glomerulopathy
  - Other causes: Trauma, dehydration (infancy), hypercoagulable states, oral contraceptives, steroid use
  - Usually RV thrombosis is unilateral (left most common), may be bilateral
  - Thromboembolic events common (especially pulmonary embolism)
- Epidemiology
  - Acute RV thrombosis
    - Predominately infants, young children, young adults
    - May resolve but commonly leads to renal atrophy
  - Chronic RV thrombosis
    - Older adults
    - Strong association with preceding renal disease
    - Associated with slowly progressive renal failure

Clinical Issues
Presentation
- Acute: Flank or abdominal pain, mass (kidney), hematuria, proteinuria
- Chronic: No direct symptoms, presents with renal failure, recurrent thromboembolism

Treatment
- Supportive measures, hemodialysis, anticoagulation (acute), thrombolysis delined through vein and artery (acute)

Prognosis
- Guarded: High level of morbidity and mortality in all reported series

Selected References
1. Kawashima A et al: CT evaluation of renovascular disease. RadioGraphics 20: 1321-40, 2000
2. Heiss SG et al: Contrast-enhanced three-dimensional fast spoiled gradient-echo renal MR imaging: Evaluation of vascular and nonvascular disease. RadioGraphics 20: 1341-52, 2000
3. Schrier RW et al: Diseases of the kidney (ed. 6). Boston, Little Brown, 1903-12, 1997

Renal Vein Tumor Extension

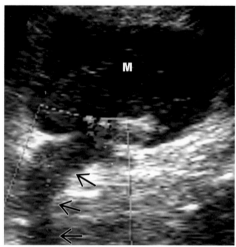

Renal vein tumor extension from RCC. Color Doppler US image from a posterolateral transducer approach shows absence of flow in the renal vein (arrows), except in tumor vessels. The primary tumor mass (M) is evident in the kidney.

Key Facts
- Synonym: Extension of tumor into renal vein (RV)
- Definition: Extension of tumor from a renal neoplasm into the RV, and possibly the inferior vena cava (IVC), occasionally right atrium
- Classic imaging appearance: RV distended by tumor with visible tumor vessels on color Doppler and tumor enhancement on contrast-enhanced CT or MRI
- Other key facts
  - RV extension occurs with renal cell carcinoma (RCC), Wilms tumor, transitional cell carcinoma, lymphoma
  - Reported incidence of RCC extension to RV 21-35%, IVC 5-10%

Imaging Findings
Best Imaging Clue
- Enhancement of RV tumor differentiates tumor and thrombus (non-enhancing)
CT Findings
- RV may be distended
- RV tumor probably not visible on non-contrast scans
- CTA: Hypodense filling defect in RV, or absence of flow (with occlusion)
- Possible "tram-track" sign of blood flow around tumor
- Enhancement of RV tumor during arterial and venous phases
- Tumor may be invisible in equilibrium phase (blood and tumor = density)
- Renal primary readily seen, enhances in arterial phase
MR Findings
- RV may be distended
- Low or intermediate signal in RV tumor on non-contrast T1 and T2 weighted images
- Low signal filling defect in RV, well seen on TOF or phase contrast MRA
- Gd-enhanced MRA does not clearly improve RV/IVC tumor visualization

Renal Vein Tumor Extension

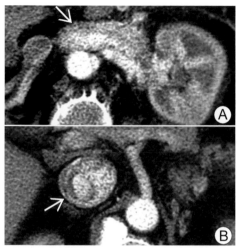

RCC tumor extension (arterial-phase contrast-enhanced CT). (A) The left renal vein (arrow) is distended by strongly enhancing tumor. (B) Tumor is seen to extend into the IVC (arrow). The superior end of the tumor (not shown) was just below the diaphragm.

- RV tumor enhancement visible on T1 weighted images follow Gd enhancement
- Renal primary readily seen, variable enhancement with Gd

Ultrasound Findings
- RV may be distended
- Tumor in RV hypoechoic or intermediate echogenicity
- RV flow void on color Doppler (absent flow with occlusion)
- Tumor vessels in RV shown with color Doppler (low PRF, high sensitivity required)
- Low resistance Doppler waveforms in tumor vessels
- Renal primary readily seen, including tumor vessels, on color Doppler

Imaging Recommendations
- CTA or MRA are best modalities for determining the presence and extent of RV tumor
- MRA superior to CT for IVC tumor extent (CT compromised by flow artifact, especially from renal veins)
- Cardiac motion may interfere with MRI visualization of tumor high in IVC or right atrium
- Color Doppler US can visualize superior extent of IVC tumor through liver "window"
- Overall accuracy of color Doppler US excellent in small children, poor in adults (RV visualization problems)

Differential Diagnosis

RV Thrombosis
- Considerable overlap in CT/MR and US findings, but
- No enhancement of thrombus on CT/MR, no tumor vessels on US
- Renal primary readily seen in cases of RV tumor extension

Renal Vein Tumor Extension

Sluggish RV Flow
- Due to extrinsic RV/IVC compression, or IVC obstruction
- Potential false positive for RV occlusion on US and non-contrast MRA

Pathology
General
- RCC is most common tumor, by far, to extend to the RV / IVC
- In cases of RV extension, RCC primary at least 4.5 cm
- IVC extension most often from the right kidney (vein shorter than left)

Gross Pathologic or Surgical Features
- Venous RCC is poorly attached and can be removed surgically with clear margins
- Both tumor and bland thrombus are present in most specimens

Staging or Grading Criteria
- RCC extension to RV and IVC graded as Robson stage IIIa

Clinical Issues
Presentation
- RV tumor extension, per se, is usually asymptomatic
- Presentation usually is that of the renal primary tumor (e.g., hematuria, mass, constitutional symptoms)
- Secondary RV thrombosis can produce acute RV occlusion symptoms

Treatment
- Surgical resection of kidney and venous tumor
- It is important to know extent of venous tumor, as this dictates surgical approach

Prognosis
- Not substantially different from stage I and II disease, much better than stage III (lymph node mets)
- > 60% 5-year survival in most series

Selected References
1. Kawashima A et al: CT evaluation of renovascular disease. RadioGraphics 20: 1321-40, 2000
2. Heiss SG et al: Contrast-enhanced three-dimensional fast spoiled gradient-echo renal MR imaging: Evaluation of vascular and nonvascular disease. RadioGraphics 20: 1341-52, 2000
3. Motzer RJ et al: Renal-cell Carcinoma. New England J Med 335: 865-75, 1996

Renal Cell Carcinoma

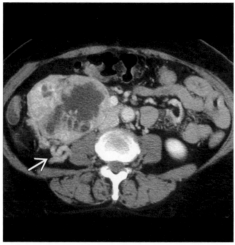

Large hypervascular mass replacing lower pole of the kidney. Tumor has extended far beyond capsule of kidney to involve retroperitoneal structures. Large collateral vessel seen posteriorly (arrow).

Key Facts
- Synonym: RCC, Hypernephroma, renal cell adenocarcinoma, clear cell carcinoma & Grawitz tumor
- Definition: Malignant renal neoplasm
- Classic imaging appearance: Vascular renal mass
- Other key facts
  - Most common primary renal tumor (30,000 new cases each year in US)
  - 2% of all cancers
  - > 50% RCCs found incidentally on CT, ultrasound or MR of abdomen
  - 5-year survival has increased to 60%

Imaging Findings
General Features
- Best imaging clue: Hypervascular renal cortical mass
- **Metastatic RCC** seen in lungs, mediastinum, bone & liver
- Extensive tumor involves adjacent organs (liver, spleen), abdominal wall
CT Findings
- NECT
  - Solid tissue density mass in 30-50 HU range, distorting normal kidney contour, extending outside kidney
  - Calcifications present in ~ 30%
- CECT
  - Hypervascular
  - **Nephrographic phase** most sensitive for tumor detection
    - Particularly small (≤ 3 cm) masses
  - **Corticomedullary phase** required for tumor extension into renal veins
    - Evaluation for hypervascular metastases
  - Helical CT improves diagnosis eliminating respiratory misregistration
MR Findings
- T1WI- most common has signal intensity between cortex and medulla

259

Renal Cell Carcinoma

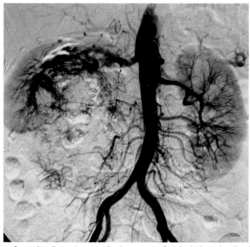

Aortogram of renal cell carcinoma, displacement of right kidney by the lower pole mass, hypervascular with tumor vascularity, collateral supply from lumbar arteries, displacement of aorta by the mass.

- T2WI – often hyperintense, similar to parenchyma
- Multiplanar capability ideal for detection of renal vein & IVC extension

Ultrasound Findings
- Primary goal to determine if mass is cystic or solid
- RCC typically have multiple septations, septal thickening, nodularity & solid components, hypoechoic or hyperechoic with majority isoechoic
- High velocity signal in Doppler ultrasound from arteriovenous shunting

Angiography Findings
- Hypervascular mass, evaluate for renal vein involvement, IVC involvement, metastases
- Guiding therapy, primarily alcohol ablation prior to surgery

Imaging Recommendations
- Multiphase CT ideal for RCC staging & preoperative planning
  - Arterial phase: Early corticomedullary phase
  - Corticomedullary phase: Enhancing renal cortex, limited medullary
  - Nephrographic phase: Full capillary level renal enhancement
  - Excretory phase: Contrast in collecting system
- 3D mapping with volume rendering ± maximum intensity projection technique ideal for preoperative staging

Differential Diagnosis
Hemorrhagic Renal Cyst
- Avascular RCC can look similar
- Differentiation usually possible with multiphase renal CT imaging
Renal Abscess
- Focal abscess can simulate necrotic tumor
- Clinical history & urinalysis distinguish abscess from RCC
Transitional Cell Carcinoma
- Tends to have calyceal invasion

Renal Cell Carcinoma

Metastases to Kidney
- Most are hypovascular
- If hypervascular, may mimic RCC

Renal Lymphoma
- Hypovascular intrarenal mass
- May have associated adenopathy

Pathology

General
- Etiology-Pathogenesis
  - From proximal convoluted tubular epithelium, usually in renal cortex
- Epidemiology
  - Most common primary renal tumor
    - 30,000 new cases each year in USA, 2% of all cancers
    - 12,000 deaths per year in USA

Microscopic Features
- Clear cell (75%), chromophilic (15%), oncocytoma (3%), collecting duct (2%)

Staging Criteria
- Several staging systems – Robson and TNM
- Robson has been the most widely recognized system
- TNM is now the most widely accepted pathologic staging system

Clinical Issues

Presentation
- Most common sign/symptom: Gross hematuria (60%)
- Classic triad: Gross hematuria, flank pain (50%) & palpable renal mass present in < 10% of cases
- Occurs with increased frequency in patients with Von Hippel-Lindau disease, tuberous sclerosis, acquired cystic renal disease & hereditary renal cell carcinoma
- Demographics: Male-to-female ratio: 2:1; age: 50-70 year olds

Treatment
- Surgery is the treatment of choice with **partial nephrectomy** more commonly used
  - CT angiography & 3D mapping preoperatively make this possible
  - Partial nephrectomy requires ≤ 5 cm tumor size
  - Peripheral location, exophytic extension and lack of vessel invasion & nodal spread also make possible
- Surgery considered worthwhile even with metastatic disease
- Preoperative embolization for larger tumors outside renal capsule
- Chemotherapy & radiation therapy have not proven of great value

Prognosis
- 5-year survival is 60%; drops to 5-10% if distant metastases present

Selected References
1. Gettman MT et al: Update on pathologic staging of renal cell carcinoma. Urology 60: 209-17, 2002
2. Sheth S et al: Current concepts in the diagnosis and management of renal cell carcinoma: Role of multidetector CT & three-dimensional CT. Radiographics 21: S237-54, 2001
3. Herts BR et al: Triphasic helical CT of the kidneys: Contribution of vascular phase scanning in patients before urologic surgery. AJR 173: 1273-7, 1999

Renal Transplant Dysfunction

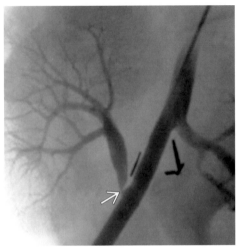

Stenosis of renal transplant artery (arrow). Typical position of stenosis at the anastomosis of the donor renal artery to the recipient external iliac artery. Note the presence of clips that may compromise MR imaging.

Key Facts
- Definition: Dysfunction of renal transplant due to renal artery stenosis
- Classic imaging appearance: Narrowing of the transplant renal artery
- Renal artery stenosis most common vascular complication, venous stenosis may also be responsible for renal dysfunction
- Stenosis in arteries proximal to transplant may cause dysfunction
- Arteriovenous fistula from biopsy may cause renal transplant dysfunction
- Differentiate anatomic dysfunction from rejection and obstruction
- Usually end-to-side anastomosis of renal artery/vein to external iliac artery/vein

Imaging Findings
General Features
- Best imaging clue: Ultrasound of the renal artery demonstrating high peak systolic velocity (>2-2.5 m/s) waveform

CT Findings
- Not usually applicable in transplants because of the need for large volumes of contrast

MR Findings
- MRI/MRA can be used to evaluate transplant
- 3D MRA may be very useful, MIP and/or MPVR techniques
- Presence of surgical clips may compromise imaging

Ultrasound Findings
- Excellent modality for evaluating vascularity of renal transplant
- Absence of arterial or venous signal prompts surgery or angiography
- Doppler exam - high peak systolic velocity waveform (2-2.5 m/s) indicates renal artery stenosis
  - Stenosis usually at anastomosis or proximal donor artery
  - Turbulence, flow reversal and spectral broadening - secondary findings
- Doppler exam - reversed diastolic flow suggests venous obstruction

Renal Transplant Dysfunction

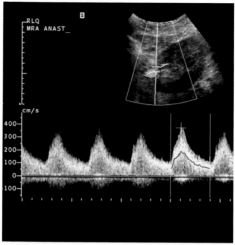

Doppler exam of renal transplant artery. Main renal artery anastomosis is being interrogated. High peak systolic velocity waveform (> 200 cm/sec) is indicatative of renal artery stenosis. Stenosis is usually at anastomosis of proximal donor artery. (Courtesy Michele Brown MD)

- Evaluate iliac artery/vein, exclude proximal lesion causing poor function
- Arteriovenous fistulas demonstrated with color flow ultrasound

Nuclear Medicine Scan Findings
- Used to assess function, Tc-99m MAG for acute tubular necrosis
- Captopril renal scans may be helpful

Angiography Findings
- Confirm ultrasound findings of arterial/venous stenosis or occlusion
- Evaluate inflow
- Used to guide therapy
- Gadolinium or CO_2 used as contrast agents when renal insufficiency

Imaging Recommendations
- Duplex, color-flow ultrasound as a screening test
- MRI/MRA, particularly in obese patients

Differential Diagnosis

Rejection vs. Acute Tubular Necrosis
- Color Doppler can be useful, but histology is required
- Resistive indices that are high suggest acute rejection

Venous Thrombosis
- Dilated vein containing thrombus
- Absent venous flow
- Reverse diastolic flow within infrarenal and transplant renal arteries

Arteriovenous Fistula
- Secondary to transplant biopsy, incidence 1-2%
- Increased systolic and diastolic flow
- Usually small and insignificant, maybe associated with hemorrhage
- If large may result in ischemia and transplant dysfunction

Obstruction
- Ultrasound used to diagnose hydronephrosis

Renal Transplant Dysfunction

- Ultrasound for diagnosis of postoperative fluid collections which may occlude ureter/vein

Pathology

General
- General Path Comments
  - Hypertension - renal ischemia – causing activation of renin angiotensin system
- Etiology-Pathogenesis
  - Predisposing factors – renal donor atherosclerosis, transplantation of pediatric kidneys into adults
  - Surgical – trauma to donor or recipient arteries, clamp injury, traction on renal vessels, suture technique
  - Atherosclerosis of recipient's iliac arteries
- Epidemiology
  - Renal artery stenosis occurs in up to 10% of renal transplants

Gross Pathologic or Surgical Features
- Intimal flaps, subintimal dissection, intimal scarring, hyperplasia

Clinical Issues

Presentation
- May be asymptomatic
- Accelerated or difficult to control hypertension, progressive renal impairment, deterioration in renal function following ACE inhibitor therapy
- Flash pulmonary edema

Natural History
- Unclear, potentially reversible cause of morbidity and graft dysfunction

Treatment
- Medical therapy: Drug intolerance is common, progressive renal failure
- Surgical therapy: Success 65-90%, risk of graft loss, ureteral injury, restenosis 12%
- Angioplasty: First line of therapy, technical success > 80%, hypertension control > 75%, renal function stable or improved > 80%, restenosis 10-33%
  - Stent placement – may improve restenosis rate
  - Treatment of iliac or aortic stenosis with angioplasty/stents

Prognosis
- Poor without therapy
- With angioplasty, good technical and clinical response can be expected

Selected References
1. Baxter GM: Ultrasound of renal transplantation. Clin Radiol 56: 802-18, 2001
2. Hohenwalter MD et al: Renal transplant evaluation with MR angiography and MR imaging. Radiographics 21: 1505-17, 2001
3. Spinosa DJ et al: Angiographic evaluation and treatment of transplant renal artery stenosis. Curr Opin Urol 11: 197-205, 2001

Fibromuscular Dysplasia, Renal

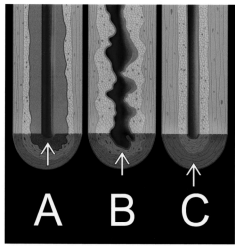

Types of fibromuscular dysplasia (FMD): (A) Intimal fibroplasias, (B) medial fibroplasias, (C) periadventitial (perimedial) fibrosis. Arrows point to abnormal layers.

Key Facts
- Definition: Dysplastic arterial wall disorder characterized by overgrowth of smooth muscle and fibrous tissue
- Classic imaging appearance
  - Serial circular ridges encroaching on the arterial lumen
  - "String-of-beads" arteriographic appearance
- Other key facts
  - Female predominance (90% in adults)
  - Principally affects renal artery (RA)

Imaging Findings
Best Imaging Clue
- Multifocal, bilateral RA stenoses, especially distal RA or hilar branches
- Appearance as above
CTA, MRA, DSA Findings
- Most common: Multifocal stenosis, ring-like ridges, or "string of beads"
- Usually distal main RA or hilar branches
- 70% bilateral, if unilateral almost always right RA
- Other appearances
  - Single focal stenosis
  - Long tapered stenosis
- Complications
  - Occlusion
  - Aneurysm (usually in post-stenotic region)
  - Dissection
  - Distal embolization
Ultrasound Findings
- Distinguishing findings seen only in cases of excellent resolution (e.g., in children)
- Visible ridges or thickening of artery wall, with or without stenosis

Fibromuscular Dysplasia, Renal

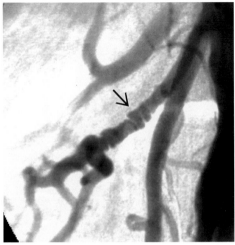

RA fibromuscular dysplasia (FMD). Multiple web-like stenoses (arrow) are seen in the distal right RA, producing a "string-of-beads" appearance. (65-year-old woman with hypertension).

- Elevated velocity and disturbed flow in areas of stenosis

Imaging Recommendations
- DSA remains the "gold standard" diagnostic modality
- MRA, CTA for noninvasive assessment, less accurate than DSA
- 3D contrast-enhanced MRA required for accurate RA diagnosis
- CTA is in evolution, multidetector technology will improve accuracy
- Visualization of the hilar RA branches is crucial (potential limitation of MRA and CTA)
- US not primary diagnostic method: Limited visualization of hilar RA branch vessels (except small children)

Differential Diagnosis

Atherosclerosis
- Does not produce concentric ridges or "string-of-beads" appearance
- Usually focal, solitary stenosis at RA origin
- Multifocal, distal RA or hilar branch stenosis uncommon

Arteritis
- Often other vessels involved
- Does not produce "string-of-pearls" appearance
- Intimal type with longer segment narrowing may appear more similar to arteritis

Pathology

General
- General Path Comments
  - Dysplastic disorder, not degenerative or inflammatory
  - Characterized by overgrowth of smooth muscle cells and fibrous tissue within arterial wall in three patterns (See "Gross Pathologic or Surgical Features" below)
  - RA predominance, carotid & iliac arteries distant 2nd & 3rd in frequency

Fibromuscular Dysplasia, Renal

- o May affect other medium-size arteries (peripheral, abdominal, cephalic)
- o Alternating zones of hyperplasia and weakening; narrowing and dilatation = "string-of-beads" appearance
- o Weakened areas may cause aneurysm formation or dissection
- Genetics
  - o Not classical genetic disorder
  - o Familial in 11% of cases
  - o Female predominance (90% of adult patients are female)
- Epidemiology
  - o 4.4% asymptomatic incidence of RA FMD in adult renal transplant donors
- Etiology-Pathogenesis
  - o Unknown

Gross Pathologic or Surgical Features
- Three principle varieties
  - o Medial fibroplasia
    - ▪ Medial layer involvement
    - ▪ 85% of cases
  - o Periadventitial (perimedial) fibrosis
    - ▪ Involvement of adventitia adjacent to media
  - o Intimal fibroplasia
    - ▪ Intimal involvement

Clinical Issues

Presentation
- Symptoms principally due to arterial stenosis/occlusion
- Renovascular hypertension and transient cerebral ischemia most common presentations
- Think of FMD in a child or young adult with hypertension, especially if female
- May present at any age, overlaps atherosclerosis age range

Treatment
- Balloon angioplasty is treatment of choice, > 95% cure/improvement of renovascular hypertension
- Surgical bypass used infrequently

Prognosis
- Guarded, slowly progressive disorder
- Long-term angioplasty and surgical results are excellent

Selected References
1.	Moore WS: Vascular surgery: a comprehensive review, ed 6. Philadelphia, WB Saunders, 142-3, 295, 306-7, 2002
2.	Papachristopoulos G et al: Breath-hold 3D MR angiography of the renal vasculature using a contrast-enhanced multiecho gradient-echo technique. Invest Radiol 34: 731-8, 1999
3.	Beregi JP et al: Fibromuscular dysplasia of the renal arteries: Comparison of helical CT angiography and arteriography. AJR 72: 27-34, 1999

267

PocketRadiologist™
Vascular
Top 100 Diagnoses

UPPER/LOWER EXTREMITY

Aberrant Right Subclavian Artery

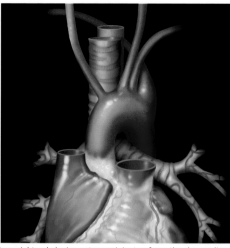

The anomalous right subclavian artery originates from the descending aorta as the last branch. It then passes obliquely cephalad and to the right, passing behind the esophagus.

Key Facts
- Definition: Congenital aortic arch anomaly
- Classic imaging appearance: Anomalous right subclavian artery originating from the descending aortic arch as the last branch
- Most common congenital anomaly of the aortic arch
- Incidence of 0.4-2.3%
- Associated with congenital heart disease in 10-15%
- Often (60%) there is dilatation of the origin of the aberrant subclavian artery referred to as a diverticulum of Kommerell

Imaging Findings
General Features
- Best imaging clue: Large vessel arising from the distal aorta and passing behind the esophagus with oblique course to the right
- Kommerell's diverticulum: Enlargement of the origin of the aberrant right subclavian
CT Findings
- Large vessel arising from the arch of the aorta and passing obliquely behind the esophagus
- Evaluate presence of airway narrowing, unlikely except for small percent of patients when the artery lies anterior to the trachea
MR Findings
- MR is the method of choice for evaluation
- Coronal SE using thin slices through the junction of the transverse and descending aorta
- Demonstrate the origin and proximal aspect of the aberrant vessel as it passes posterior to the esophagus
Chest Radiograph Findings
- Lateral view demonstrates indentation of the posterior aspect of the trachea

Aberrant Right Subclavian Artery

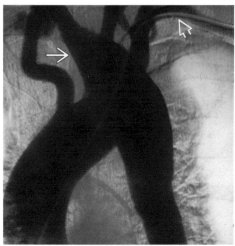

Aberrant right subclavian artery arises in distal aorta and courses obliquely to the right. Diverticulum of Kommerell (arrow) is the dilation at the origin of the subclavian. Note the catheter (open arrow) has been placed via the left subclavian artery.

- Frontal view may show widening of right paratracheal soft tissue
- If aneurysmal subclavian there may be prominence of the left mediastinum

Esophagogram
- Indentation of the posterior wall of the esophagus by an aberrant right subclavian artery

Imaging Recommendations
- MRI helpful to delineate vascular anatomy
- Multidetector CT with reconstruction is alternative

Differential Diagnosis

Right Aortic Arch with Aberrant Left Subclavian
- Left subclavian arises from the descending aorta
- May be posterior indentation in barium-filled esophagus
- Trachea may be displaced anteriorly
- Also may have a diverticulum of Kommerell of the left subclavian artery
- Rarely associated with congenital heart disease

Double Aortic Arch
- Persistence of both fetal arches
- Bilateral indentations of esophagus on AP view as well posterior
- Right carotid and subclavian arise from the right-sided arch
- Left common carotid and subclavian from left arch

Pathology

General
- General Path Comments
  - Passes behind the esophagus
  - May cause dysphagia, but usually asymptomatic
  - Rarely may lie anterior to the trachea (5%)

Aberrant Right Subclavian Artery

- Embryology-Anatomy
  - Disappearance of the right fourth aortic arch and persistence of the normally disappearing right dorsal arch
  - Break in the hypothetic double aortic arch between the right common carotid artery and the right subclavian artery
  - The right ductus is obliterated
  - Right subclavian can arise directly from the descending aorta or can arise from an aortic diverticulum (Kommerell)
- Epidemiology
  - Most common congenital anomaly of aortic arch
  - Incidence of 0.4%-2.3%
  - Congenital heart disease present in 10-15% of cases
  - Tetralogy of Fallot
  - Coarctation of aorta
  - In coarctation if the aberrant right subclavian arises distal to the coarctation, it serves as a major collateral

Clinical Issues
Presentation
- Usually asymptomatic because a vascular ring is not intact
- Only 5% have symptoms secondary to airway or esophageal compression
  - Symptoms may develop when artery is tortuous or aneurysmal
Treatment
- Surgery rarely indicated
- Most commonly an incidental finding

Selected References
1.   Donnelly LF: Aberrant subclavian arteries: cross-sectional imaging findings in infants and children referred for evaluation of extrinsic airway compression. AJR 178: 1269-74, 2002
2.   Lund GK et al: Magnetic resonance imaging of congenital anomalies of the thoracic aorta. In: Taveras J and Ferrucci J. Radiology Vol 2, Chap 31A, 2001
3.   Strife JL: Cardiovascular system. In: Kirks DR, ed. Practical pediatric radiology. 3rd ed.: 511-613, 1998

Subclavian Vein Thrombosis

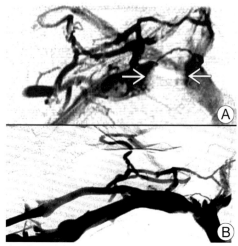

Acute effort thrombosis. (A) DSA showing a short-segment occlusion of the subclavian vein (arrows) multiple collaterals present. (B) DSA after thrombolysis. Some residual stenosis is present, which subsequently was corrected with angioplasty, note decrease in collaterals.

Key Facts
- Synonym: Subclavian thrombophlebitis
- Definition: Thrombus formation in the subclavian vein, usually accompanied by axillary vein thrombosis
- Common cause: Indwelling venous catheters, thoracic outlet syndrome
- 40% incidence of persistent venous insufficiency symptoms
- Imaging findings change from acute to subacute/chronic phases

Imaging Findings
Best Diagnostic Finding (Acute)
- Subclavian vein occlusion with extensive collateralization
- Thrombus "filling defect" in vein lumen with flow around thrombus
CTA, MRA, DSA Findings
- Acute
  - Thrombus = filling defect
  - Contrast flow around thrombus
    - "Tram-track" appearance, long axis views
    - "Target" appearance, short axis views
  - Distended veins distal to thrombus
  - Extensive collateral network
  - Perivascular inflammatory changes on MRI
- Subacute and chronic
  - Variable thrombus lysis and vein recanalization
Ultrasound Findings
- Acute
  - Vein markedly distended
  - Hypoechoic, homogeneous thrombus
  - Possible small flow streams around and through thrombus

Subclavian Vein Thrombosis

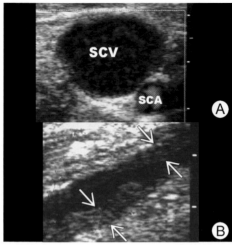

(A) Acute subclavian thrombosis. The subclavian vein (SCV) is markedly distended as compared with the subclavian artery (SCA) and is filled with low-echogenic, homogeneous thrombus. (B) Chronic subclavian thrombosis (4 months by history). The vein wall (arrows) is thick and irregular.

- Subacute
  - Increased thrombus echogenicity/heterogeneity
  - Shrinkage of thrombus, decreased vein size
- Chronic stage
  - Possible return to normal appearance
  - Scarred veins
    - Localized or diffuse wall thickening, plaque-like scars, webs
    - Variable vein caliber: Normal, stenotic, or small fibrotic vein with or without blood flow

Imaging Recommendations
- Ultrasound is principal diagnostic method, but
  - Ultrasound limited to distal subclavian vein and arm veins
  - Ultrasound accuracy is unknown
- CTA and MRV
  - Appear accurate, but subject to thrombus - mimicking flow artifacts
  - Contrast enhanced MRV appears superior to non-contrast MRV
  - Determine cause of extrinsic venous compression
- Thoracic outlet obstruction: Use CTA, MRV or contrast venography

Differential Diagnosis
Lymphatic Obstruction (Lymphedema)
- Venous system normal
Extrinsic Venous Compression
- Location varies from superior vena cava to axillary vein
- Thrombosis (secondary to stasis) may or may not be present
- Usual cause: Lymphadenopathy
- Other causes: Pancoast lung cancer, scarring (e.g., post radiation)
Thoracic Outlet Syndrome (See "Subclavian Stenosis/Occlusion")
- Subclavian vein compressed between ribs 1 & 2 and scalene muscles

Subclavian Vein Thrombosis

- Intermittent arm pain/swelling due to venous congestion
- Possible arterial ischemia and brachial plexus neuropathy

Pathology
General
- Underlying cause usually present; often combination of factors
- Inflammation
  - May **cause** thrombosis or **result from** thrombosis
  - Perivascular inflammation may be seen with MRI
- Thrombus evolves with time (see "Venous Thrombosis, Acute/Subacute")
- Genetics
  - Deficiency or abnormality of factor VII cause recurrent thrombosis
- Embryology-Anatomy
  - Cervical rib and other variants can contribute to thoracic outlet obstruction and effort thrombosis
- Etiology-Pathogenesis
  - Venous catheters and pacemaker electrodes (intimal injury)
  - Other vein injury: Trauma, caustic infusion (e.g., heroin)
  - Stasis (e.g., from lymphadenopathy, tumors, scar)
  - Hypercoagulable states
- Effort thrombosis
  - Subclavian/axillary vein thrombosis presenting within 24 hrs after unusual or prolonged physical activity
  - Frequently seen in bodybuilders and other athletes
  - Medical emergency to prevent debilitation from permanent subclavian occlusion (40-70% long-term symptoms)

Clinical Issues
Presentation
- Upper extremity swelling
- Arm pain varying from dull ache to severe discomfort
- Visible collaterals, shoulder and thorax
- Palpable tender axillary "cord" (thrombosed axillary vein)
- Associated pulmonary emboli 5-15% of subclavian/axillary thrombosis
Treatment
- Anticoagulation and supportive measures initially
  - Anticoagulation, thrombolysis or thrombectomy
- Aggressive therapy recommended for effort thrombosis
- Relieve extrinsic venous compression, if present
- Angioplasty or venous bypass surgery for chronic symptomatic occlusion
Prognosis
- Guarded
- Venous insufficiency after subclavian thrombosis
  - Overall, at least 40% of patients, range mild to severe
  - After effort thrombosis, 40-70% incidence

Selected References
1. Marinella MA et al: Spectrum of upper-extremity deep venous thrombosis in a community teaching hospital. Heart Lung 29: 113-7, 2000
2. Browse NL et al: Diseases of the Veins, London, Arnold/Oxford Press, 689-707, 1999
3. Haire WD et al: Limitations of magnetic resonance imaging and ultrasound-directed (duplex) scanning in the diagnosis of subclavian vein thrombosis. J Vasc Surg 13: 391-3, 1991

Subclavian Stenosis/Occlusion

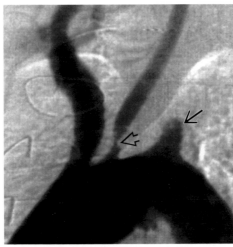

Digital subtraction angiogram showing occlusion of the left subclavian artery (arrow). The patient was asymptomatic with respect to this finding, which was discovered in the course of carotid sonography. A high-grade stenosis of the left common carotid artery (open arrow) was also discovered sonographically.

Key Facts
- Synonyms: Subclavian obstruction, subclavian occlusive disease
- Definition: Subclavian artery (SCA) luminal narrowing (stenosis) or occlusion
- Classic imaging appearance: Narrowing or obstruction of the SCA lumen
- Other key facts
  - 85% of atherosclerosis-related cases occur in the left SCA
  - Most common atherosclerosis locations
    - SCA origin
    - Just proximal to vertebral artery origin
  - Associated with the vertebral-to-subclavian steal

Imaging Findings
General Features
- Best imaging clue: Focal narrowing or occlusion of the SCA
CTA, MRA or DSA Findings
- Post-stenotic dilatation (severe stenosis)
- Long, smoothly tapered stenosis with dissection
- Reversed vertebral artery flow (subclavian steal)
- Collateralized vessels in the chest wall and shoulder
- Soft-tissue masses or scar (if obstructed by extrinsic compression)
- Vessel compression at the thoracic outlet, possibly with post stenotic aneurysm (thoracic outlet syndrome)
Duplex Ultrasound Findings
- Absence of flow in occluded segment
- Elevated flow velocity in stenosis (peak systolic velocity $\geq$ 300 cm/sec)
- Post-stenotic flow disturbance
- Damped Doppler waveforms in SCA/axillary artery distal to obstruction
- Reversed or to-and-fro flow in ipsilateral vertebral artery

Subclavian Stenosis/Occlusion

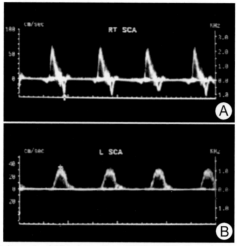

Doppler US diagnosis of SCA obstruction. (A) Right SCA: Normal triphasic Doppler waveforms (forward, reverse, forward). (B) Post-stenotic left SCA: Monophasic waveforms with slow acceleration to peak (pulsus tardus), and low flow velocity overall (pulsus parvus). Peak systolic velocity 70 cm/sec right and 35 cm/sec left.

Imaging Recommendations
- Sonography to diagnose or confirm SCA occlusive disease
- MRA, CTA, or DSA for pre-treatment assessment
- MRI or CT to diagnose extrinsic SCA compression (tumor, scar)
- Duplex Ultrasound, CTA, MRA to diagnose the thoracic outlet syndrome

Differential Diagnosis
Thoracic Outlet Syndrome
- Arm pain due to compression of the neurovascular bundle (subclavian artery and vein, brachial plexus) at the thoracic outlet
- Symptoms most often from brachial plexus compression
- Symptoms also from intermittent occlusion of the subclavian artery
- Boundaries of thoracic outlet: Clavicle and first ribs, anterior and posterior scalene muscles
- Vascular laboratory diagnosis: Changes in spectral Doppler waveforms or arm blood pressure in response to provocative arm and head maneuvers (e.g., Adson maneuver)
- CTA/MRA diagnosis: Compression of SCA at thoracic outlet, possible post stenotic aneurysm (diagnostic feature)
Embolization/Iatrogenic
- 30% upper extremity ischemia is embolic
- 30% upper extremity ischemia iatrogenic (e.g., arterial puncture, catheterization, hemodialysis access)

Pathology
General
- Atherosclerosis – causes about 30% of upper extremity ischemia cases, typically in elderly and typically asymptomatic

Subclavian Stenosis/Occlusion

- Arterial dissection (usually from trauma or extending from the aortic arch)
- Neoplastic compression/invasion (especially Pancoast lung tumor)
- Trauma (blunt or penetrating, iatrogenic)
- Scar (e.g., post radiation, fibrosing mediastinitis)
- Thoracic outlet syndrome
- Fibromuscular dysplasia
- Vasculitis (e.g., Takayasu's disease, giant cell arteritis)
- Congenital absence of the SCA (rare)
- Anatomy
  o Potential for traumatic injury with clavicle fracture
  o Compression at thoracic outlet
  o Unique vertebral artery anatomy enables vertebral steal collateral flow to SCA (union of the two VAs at the foramen magnum)

Clinical Issues
Diagnostic Features
- Diminished upper extremity pulses ipsilateral to SCA obstruction
- 20 to 30 mmHg arm blood pressure difference is diagnostic
- Cold, blanched extremity with acute occlusion
Presentation
- Atherosclerosis, in elderly: Often an incidental, asymptomatic finding on physical examination or Doppler ultrasound
- Upper extremity claudication (exercise-induced ischemic pain)
- Acute arm ischemia
- Vertebrobasilar ischemic symptoms (subclavian steal)
- Distal upper extremity embolization (atherosclerosis)
- Intermittent arm, shoulder and neck pain (thoracic outlet compression)
- Myocardial ischemia post left internal mammary coronary artery bypass and subsequent SCA origin stenosis
Treatment
- No treatment for asymptomatic cases
- Angioplasty/stenting, treatment of choice
- Arterial bypass surgery for severe ischemia (e.g., axillo-axillary bypass)
- Thoracic outlet decompression surgery
Prognosis
- Atherosclerotic SCA obstruction usually remains asymptomatic, but arm claudication or posterior fossa symptoms may develop as atherosclerosis progresses
- Symptomatic dissection: Requires an angioplasty or bypass surgery
- Fibromuscular dysplasia and vasculitis are progressive
- Variable prognosis for thoracic outlet compression symptoms

Selected References
1. Edwards JM et al: Assessment of upper extremity arteries. In Zwiebel WJ (ed): Introduction to Vascular Ultrasonography, 4th Ed. Philadelphia, W.B. Saunders, 167-76, 2000
2. Van Grimberge F et al: Role of magnetic resonance in the diagnosis of subclavian steal syndrome. Magn Reson Imaging 12: 339-42, 2000
3. Taneja K et al: Occlusive arterial disease of the upper extremity: Colour Doppler as a screening technique and for assessment of distal circulation. Radiology 40: 226-9, 1996

Dialysis AVF

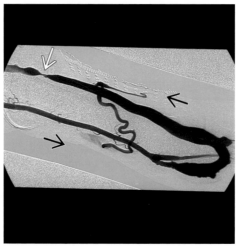

Digital subtraction angiogram of a forearm dialysis fistula. Flow is through the radial artery, there is then an anastomosis with a vein and flow is then back up the cephalic vein (black arrows show the direction of flow). White arrow demonstrates a common problem, a venous stenosis.

Key Facts
- Synonyms: Autogenous arteriovenous (AV) fistula, Brescia-Cimino AV fistula, brachiobasilic AV fistula, brachiocephalic fistula
- Definition: Surgically constructed fistula between an artery and vein for dialysis access
- Classic imaging appearance: Arteriogram, or direct puncture and fistulogram; direct arterial communication with vein
- Longest lasting and most dependable type of dialysis access if it can be established
  - Unfortunately difficult to construct, not possible in up to 65% of patients
  - Failures common in elderly and diabetic patients
  - However, once established has a primary patency of 70% at one year, and 75% patency rate at 4 years
  - In US, only about 20% have AV fistula, goal is at least 50%

Imaging Findings
General Features
- Best imaging clue: Connection between artery and vein usually in forearm, but fistulas may also be placed in the proximal upper extremity

CT Findings
- Not usually used for imaging of AV fistulas

MR Findings
- Not widely used for imaging fistulas
- MRI study of fistula should use gadolinium, increased signal-to-noise
- May be used to image the central veins if there is evidence of central venous stenosis
- MR venogram may be used in selected patients to evaluate size and patency of forearm and upper arm veins prior to surgical construction of fistula

Dialysis AVF

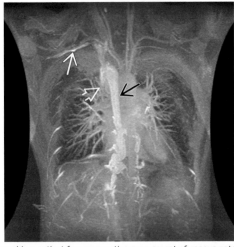

MRV performed in a patient for preoperative assessment of venous patency. Patient had previous dialysis catheters. Both subclavian veins are occluded with short, diseased segment on right (white arrow), SVC occluded (white open arrow), azygos collateral (black arrow). Demonstrates value of pre-procedure imaging.

Ultrasound Findings
- May be used in preoperative planning to evaluate the size and patency of forearm and upper arm veins
- May be used to noninvasively assess the venous flow and to look for stenoses within the venous outflow
- Not optimal for examining the central veins

Venography Findings
- Gold standard for evaluation of the preoperative planning of an AV fistula
  - Evaluates the size, position and patency of the venous system of forearm, upper arm and central veins
  - Important for patients with previously failed access, or with difficult to evaluate veins (obese patients)
- Primary evaluation of poorly maturing fistula or of functioning fistula which begins to show evidence of failing

Imaging Recommendations
- Ultrasound is the least expensive way to evaluate venous system preoperatively, not optimal for evaluating central veins
- MR venography can be excellent for central veins and can be used to evaluate arm venous system; needs to be carefully monitored to make sure that appropriate information is obtained
  - Well suited for patients with allergic reactions to contrast
- Contrast venography allows preoperative evaluation of the venous system
  - Allows for percutaneous therapy of a failing, or poorly maturing fistula

Differential Diagnosis
Dialysis Graft
- Placement of synthetic tube, usually polytetrafluoroethylene (PTFE, Gore-Tex)
- Graft may also be placed in upper thigh

- Graft is placed between artery and vein, often in a looped configuration in either forearm or in upper arm
- Unusual graft is across upper chest from axillary artery on one side to axillary vein on contralateral side

Pathology
General
- General Path Comments
  - With connection between the artery and the vein, the arterial pressure/flow is transmitted into the vein
  - Dilatation of the vein
  - Hypertrophy of the vein wall
  - Usually takes at least 6 weeks to develop sufficient size and thickness of wall to allow repeated venipuncture for dialysis
- Anatomy
  - Brescia-Cimino: Connection between radial artery and cephalic vein
    - Side-to-side, side of artery to side of vein
    - Arterial end-to-side, end of artery to side of vein
    - Venous end-to-side, end of vein to side of artery
    - End-to-end, end of artery to end of vein
    - Most common is side-to-side anastomosis

Clinical Issues
Presentation
- Venous stenosis
  - Dysfunctional dialysis
  - Arm swelling
Natural History
- If becomes functional may last for years
- If venous or arterial stenosis develops, the fistula may be treated with percutaneous methods
- May not become functional because too many draining veins, and a single vein does not become dominate
Treatment
- Angioplasty for venous stenoses
- Stents used very occasionally for venous stenosis
- If graft does not mature because of too many venous outflows, embolization of venous branches, or surgical ligation can be performed
Prognosis
- Angioplasty may need to be repeated every few months, often after several angioplasties, the vein will tend to remain patent for a longer period

Selected References
1. Sands JJ et al: The role of color flow Doppler ultrasound in dialysis access. Semin Nephrol 22: 195-201, 2002
2. Cavagna E et al: Failing hemodialysis arteriovenous fistula and percutaneous treatment: Imaging with CT, MRI, and digital subtraction angiography. Cardiovasc Intervent Radiol 23: 262-5,2000
3. Schwab SJ et al: NKF DOQI clinical practice guidelines for hemodialysis vascular access. Am J Kidney Dis 30: 150-91, 1997

Catheter Caused Venous Occlusion

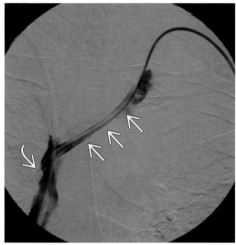

Dialysis catheter placed from the left jugular vein. Although the catheter was initially placed with the tip in the superior vena cava, the catheter has pulled back so that the tip is against the side of the superior vena cava (curved arrow). Clot has developed along the catheter (arrows); this led to arm and neck swelling.

Key Facts
- Synonym: Iatrogenic superior vena cava syndrome (if SVC involved)
- Definition: Thrombosis of the major venous structures, primarily in the upper extremities, although this can also occur in the lower extremities if catheter is placed via femoral vein
- Classic imaging appearance: Occlusion of the vein, may be with acute thrombus, or more chronic with narrowing of the vein
- Most common cause of thoracic outlet syndrome
- Usually caused by large catheters such as dialysis or pheresis catheters
- May be caused by smaller catheters, particularly if the patient has an underlying mild thoracic outlet pathology

Imaging Findings
General Features
- Best imaging clue: Thrombosis of a major vein after or during the time that a catheter has been placed

CT Findings
- CECT
  - There will be enlarged collaterals on the chest, shoulder, neck
  - Thrombosis in major vein where catheter is placed or has been placed
  - Presence of catheter

MR Findings
- Large collaterals in chest, shoulder, neck
- Thrombosis in major vein where catheter is placed or has been placed
- Presence of catheter

Ultrasound Findings
- Demonstrate thrombus in the major vein associated with catheter
- Even if thrombus is not identified, Doppler flow studies will show lack of flow and no respiratory variation

Catheter Caused Venous Occlusion

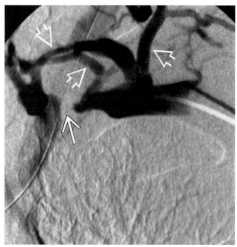

Chronic occlusion of the left subclavian vein due to previous dialysis catheter. Occlusion of the subclavian (arrow) has caused the development of multiple collaterals (open arrows). The development of such collaterals occurs relatively rapidly and may keep patient from being severely symptomatic.

Venography Findings
- Best way to visualize the venous flow, and the development of collaterals
- Provides guidance for percutaneous procedures

Imaging Recommendations
- Ultrasound is usually sufficient to make a diagnosis of thrombosis
- If therapy is contemplated, then venography will be needed to guide therapy

Differential Diagnosis

Thoracic Outlet Syndrome (Paget-Schroetter Syndrome)
- Mechanical cause for stenosis or occlusion of the subclavian vein
  - Cause of compression
    - Clavicle and subclavius muscle
    - Exostosis of first rib
    - Cervical rib

Pathology

General
- General Path Comments
  - Caused by irritation of the vein by the indwelling catheter
- Etiology-Pathogenesis
  - Intimal hyperplasia develops from the chronic irritation of the catheter
  - Stenosis develops due to the intimal hyperplasia, and then thrombosis occurs when stenosis become severe enough to restrict flow
- Epidemiology
  - Patients with indwelling catheters
    - The larger the catheter higher the likelihood of occlusion
    - Patients with dialysis catheters are at higher risk than patients with smaller catheters such as PICC lines or ports

Catheter Caused Venous Occlusion

- o Subclavian catheters are most likely to cause problems
  - Problems occur in left subclavian catheters > right subclavian catheters > left internal jugular catheter > right subclavian catheters
  - All catheters and particularly large dialysis catheters should be placed via the right internal jugular vein whenever possible
- o Patients who are hypercoagulable are more prone to thrombosis
  - Lupus anticoagulant, factor V Leiden, malignancy

Clinical Issues

Presentation
- Relatively acute swelling of the arm and neck
- If the superior vena cava is involved, then the swelling will be bilateral and the patient will have a superior vena cava syndrome
  - o Bilateral neck and arm swelling
  - o Facial swelling
  - o Mental status changes due to brain edema

Natural History
- As the collaterals develop, the arm and neck swelling may resolve
  - o Arm swelling will commonly recur if the arm is being actively used

Treatment
- Anticoagulation and arm elevation are conservative measures
- If the patient no longer requires the catheter, it should be removed
- If the patient requires continued catheter use, then if possible the patient should be managed conservatively
- Taking the catheter out and placing it in another vein places a second vein at risk
- If very symptomatic then a course of catheter-directed thrombolysis should be considered, followed by anticoagulation
- If severely symptomatic (phlegmasia cerulea dolens) thrombolysis should be initiated if possible and the catheter will probably require removal
- Some authors advocate low-dose Coumadin in patients with malignancy

Prognosis
- Commonly collaterals will form which will improve the symptoms and the catheter can remain in place
- Thrombolysis is generally successful in removing clot and improving the symptoms

Selected References
1. Kommareddy A: Upper extremity deep venous thrombosis. Semin Thromb Hemost 28: 89-99, 2002
2. Ratcliffe M et al: Thrombosis, markers of thrombotic risk, indwelling central venous catheters and antithrombotic prophylaxis using low-dose warfarin in subjects with malignant disease. Clinic and Lab Haematology 21: 353-7, 1999
3. Trerotola SO: Interventional radiology in central venous stenosis and occlusion. Semin in Interv Radiol 11: 291-304, 1994

Thoracic Outlet Syndrome, Venous

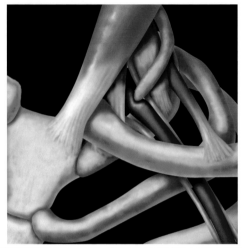

Anatomy of the thoracic outlet area. The vein passes between the clavicle, and the first rib and is surrounded by the subclavius muscle, and the anterior scalenus and the middle scalenus muscles. Compression can caused by cervical rib, or by muscular or ligamentous impingement.

Key Facts
- Synonym: Paget-Schroetter syndrome
- Definition: Compression of the axillosubclavian vein by muscular / skeletal or ligamentous structures
- Structures responsible for compression
  - Compression of subclavian vein by clavicle and subclavius muscle
  - Compression by exostosis of first rib
  - Compression by cervical rib
- Classic imaging appearance: Narrowing of the axillosubclavian vein with extension maneuvers

Imaging Findings
General Features
- Narrowing of axillosubclavian vein, may be only evident on stress views
- Collateral veins may develop if there is significant narrowing or if thrombosis develops

CT Findings
- CECT
  - Requires stress views of subclavian vein with 3D reconstruction
  - Filling of collaterals in chest wall may be present particularly if thrombosis has occurred

MR Findings
- MRV
  - Requires stress views of subclavian vein
  - Collateral veins present in chest walls

Ultrasound
- Difficult to evaluate central vein
- Abnormal flow in vein, lack of respiratory variation with stress views
- Particularly marked if thrombosis is present

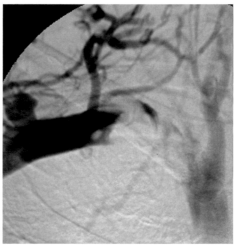

Thirty year old UPS driver presented in early January following a busy holiday delivery schedule with a history of one week of right arm swelling. DSA study demonstrates thrombus involving subclavian vein with the development of collaterals. No history of any type of catheter in major vein.

Venography
- Venogram performed from antecubital approach
- Evaluation of the veins of the upper arm and central veins
- If central vein appears normal with the arm in neutral position then perform stress views
- Stress views: The arm abducted and the head turned away from the arm being studied (Addison maneuver)
- Alternatively ask patients to perform whatever maneuvers will reproduce their symptoms

Imaging Recommendations
- Ultrasound to evaluate vein
- Venography for better evaluation and to guide therapy
  - Venography should be performed in both neutral and with provocative maneuvers (if the vein is not thrombosed)

Differential Diagnosis
History of Previous Central Line
History of Pacemaker Line
Malignant Encasement of Vein
Trauma

Pathology
General
- Anatomy
  - Compression of the subclavian vein as it passes between the clavicle and subclavius muscle anteriorly and the first rib and scalenus anticus muscle posteriorly
- Etiology-Pathogenesis

Thoracic Outlet Syndrome, Venous

- o Congenital predisposition but may be aggravated by hypertrophy of the subclavius and scalenus muscles
  - Weight lifters, surfers
- o Congenital bands and ligamentous structures
- o Bony abnormality
  - Cervical rib, exostosis of first rib, rib fractures
- o Hypercoagulable states may lead to thrombolysis
  - Protein C deficiency, protein S deficiency, antithrombin III deficiency, anticardiolipin antibody, congenital plasminogen deficiency, dysplasminogenemia, lupus anticoagulant, factor V Leiden
- Epidemiology
  - o More common in younger patients, average age 31 years
  - o More common in males, 2:1 over females

Clinical Issues

Presentation
- Pain, or heaviness of the arm particularly when raising arm over head
- Less commonly, swelling of arm (unless thrombosis has occurred)
- Younger, physically active
- Strenuous or repetitive activity before onset of symptoms

Natural History
- May progress to thrombosis
- Commonly symptoms persist, made worse with activity

Treatment
- Venography to diagnose the problem
- Subsequent surgical correction of the anatomic abnormality
- Anticoagulation
- Stenting should be avoided and is definitely not indicated until after surgical decompression

Prognosis
- Following surgery, 93% patency rate at 3 years has been reported

Selected References
1. Kommareddy A: Upper extremity deep venous thrombosis. Semin Thromb Hemost 28: 89-99, 2002
2. Machleder HI: Thrombolytic therapy and surgery for primary axillosubclavian vein thrombosis: current approach. Semin Vasc Surg 9: 46-9, 1996
3. Trerotola SO: Interventional radiology in central venous stenosis and occlusion. Semin in Interv Radiol 11: 291-304, 1994

Lower Extremity Arterial Trauma

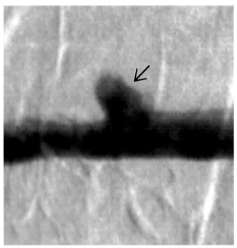

DSA of superficial femoral artery pseudoaneurysm (arrow), status post penetrating trauma. The surrounding hematoma was 4 times larger, as seen with US.

Key Facts
- Definition: Arterial injury from violent or iatrogenic trauma
- Classic imaging appearance
  - Arterial laceration, dissection, occlusion or intimal flap
  - Possible hematoma, pseudoaneurysm, or arteriovenous fistula (AVF)
- Other key facts
  - Suspect arterial injury with any penetrating trauma within 5 cm of major thigh vessels or at any location below the knee or calf
  - Vascular trauma much more frequent with penetrating injury (36%) than with blunt trauma (1%)
  - Common femoral artery frequent site of iatrogenic injury

Imaging Findings
DSA Findings
- "Gold standard" for imaging traumatized vessels
- Direct visualization of arterial lumen, revealing laceration, transection, stenosis, occlusion, dissection, pseudoaneurysm, AVF
CT Findings
- Contrast enhancement required, multidetector CTA state-of-art
- Image reformation very helpful, but review of source images also recommended
- Focal enlargement or irregularity of lumen suggests laceration
- Stenosis: Dissection, arterial spasm, extrinsic compression
- Eccentric lumen or tapered stenosis with dissection - may visualize occluded false lumen (long, eccentric filling void) in larger vessels
- Focal intraluminal defect and possible stenosis with intimal flap
- Occlusion: Arterial injury or extrinsic compression
- Localized extraluminal flow in transection and pseudoaneurysm
- Early draining vein and arteriovenous tract with AV fistula
- Hematoma/soft-tissue edema, possible fracture or joint injury
- Extravasation of contrast into soft-tissue

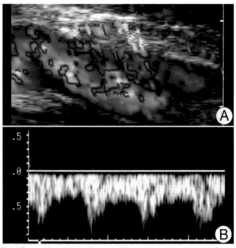

US of superficial femoral artery AVF caused by penetrating trauma. (A) Color Doppler shows marked turbulence and soft-tissue vibration at fistula site. (B) Doppler shows turbulent, pulsatile flow in draining vein.

MR Findings
- Analogous to CTA
- TOF and phase contrast images subject to artifacts
- Contrast-enhanced, 3D CTA for accurate arterial trauma evaluation

Ultrasound Findings
- Analogous to CTA
- Direct visualization of arterial defects, pseudoaneurysm, AVF
- High-velocity flow in stenosis, no flow in occlusion
- Damped Doppler waveforms distal to severe stenosis or occlusion
- Focal, severe arterial turbulence with intimal flap
- Turbulent, high-velocity venous flow in AVF

CTA, US, MRA Comparison
- CTA
  - Quick and accurate method for vascular evaluation
  - Defines scope of soft-tissue injury, hematoma
  - Identifies concomitant bone or joint injury
- Color Doppler US
  - Accurate, convenient (bedside), cost effective
  - Requires technical competence and experience
  - Cannot be used in areas of soft-tissue destruction/laceration
- Contrast enhanced, 3D MRA
  - Accurate, but more time consuming than CTA
  - May be cumbersome in acute trauma setting
  - More suitable for subacute examination

Imaging Recommendations
- Strong indication of acute arterial injury, especially if unstable
  - DSA with radiologic intervention (preferred) or surgical exploration
- Uncertain arterial injury, acute but stable
  - Investigate with CTA, US
  - Radiologic intervention (preferred) or surgical repair

Lower Extremity Arterial Trauma

- Uncertain arterial injury, subacute or chronic
  - Investigate with CTA, US or MRA
  - Radiologic intervention (preferred) or surgical repair

Differential Diagnosis
Hematoma/Contusion Without Arterial Injury
- Intact arteries
- No extraluminal blood flow (pseudoaneurysm/AVF)

Pathology
General
- Although arterial injury is more common with penetrating trauma, injury may occur with contusion only
- Delayed recognition of arterial trauma may have serious consequences

Clinical Issues
Presentation
- Acute iatrogenic trauma
  - Ecchymosis
  - Post-procedural hematoma
  - Pulsatile mass: Pseudoaneurysm
  - Audible bruit: Stenosis, intimal flap, dissection, AVF
  - Palpable thrill: AVF
  - Diminished peripheral pulses/ABI: Stenosis or occlusion, AVF
  - Cold, pale extremity: Major arterial occlusion
- Acute violent trauma
  - As above, plus
    - Open lower extremity wound
    - Possible expanding hematoma
- Subacute, chronic trauma
  - Findings as in acute, but stable
  - Possible claudication, delayed arterial rupture (pseudoaneurysm), high output heart failure or chronic venous congestion (AVF)
- Acute lower extremity fractures
  - Infrequent cause of vascular injury
  - Arterial imaging needed for diminished peripheral pulses, abnormal ankle brachial index (ABI), or severe soft-tissue crush/contusion

Precaution
- Normal peripheral pulses and ABI usually exclude lower extremity arterial injury, if there are no other findings (e.g., bruit), but it is argued that all major soft-tissue injuries (including contusion) warrant CTA, MRA or US assessment for occult vascular damage

Treatment
- Radiologic intervention is preferred over surgical arterial repair (less traumatic, faster recovery, lower cost)

Selected References
1. Soto JA et al: Focal arterial injuries of the proximal extremities: Helical CT arteriography as the initial method of diagnosis. Radiology 218(1): 188-94, 2001
2. Li WJ et al: MR angiography of the vascular tree from the aorta to the foot: Combining two-dimensional time-of-flight and three-dimensional contrast-enhanced imaging. J Magn Reson Imaging 12: 884-9,2000
3. Anderson RJ et al: Penetrating extremity trauma: Identification of patients at high-risk requiring arteriography. J Vasc Surg 11: 544-8, 1990

Popliteal Entrapment

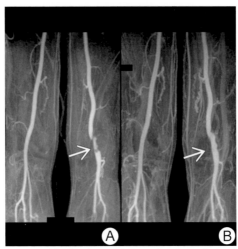

Popliteal entrapment. (A) MRA obtained during active plantar flexion demonstrates focal stenosis (arrow) of popliteal artery due to fibrous band found at surgery. (B) MRA obtained during dorsiflexion shows ectasia of popliteal artery (arrow).

Key Facts
- Synonym(s): Popliteal entrapment syndrome
- Definition: Intermittent claudication induced by compression of popliteal artery between musculoskeletal structures
- Classic imaging appearance
  - Medial deviation of the popliteal artery in the popliteal region
  - Stenosis/compression of the mid popliteal artery during prolonged plantar flexion
- Most commonly caused by compression from the medial head of the gastrocnemius muscle (74%)
- Usually presents in healthy, athletic males complaining of claudication syndrome in the absence of atherosclerosis
- Combined functional and anatomic imaging required
  - MRA or angiography in neutral position, dorsiflexion, and plantar flexion
  - MRI for anatomic definition of gastrocnemius, soleus, and popliteus muscles

Imaging Findings
General Features
- Best imaging clue: Medial deviation of popliteal artery during prolonged planter flexion with associated stenosis
CT Findings
- NECT: Limited role due to difficulty in identifying popliteal artery
- CECT
  - CTA useful for delineating the popliteal artery
  - Soft tissue contrast less well suited for demonstrating muscular anatomy than MRI
MR Findings
- T1WI: Particularly well suited for demonstrating the anatomic variants of the gastrocnemius muscle and popliteal muscle

Popliteal Entrapment

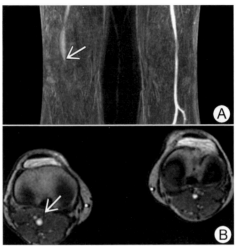

(A) CE-MRA shows complete occlusion of right popliteal artery during plantar flexion (arrow). (B) Gradient echo image demonstrates fibrous/muscular band anterior to the right popliteal artery (arrow). Image from left leg shows normal relationship of popliteal artery and vein to gastrocnemius muscle.

- Findings include
  - Popliteal artery deviates medially around the medial head of the gastrocnemius muscle
  - Medial head of gastrocnemius muscle arises laterally from the femoral condyle
  - Popliteal artery may be trapped by a lateral slip of the medial head of the gastrocnemius muscle
  - The popliteal muscle or a deep fibrous band compresses popliteal artery
- T2WI: May be helpful for identifying and characterizing other masses that may occur in the popliteal fossa
- Contrast-enhanced MRA
  - MR angiogram in neutral position demonstrates normal artery or narrowing and medial deviation of midportion of popliteal artery
  - MRA may demonstrate post-stenotic dilatation involving popliteal artery
  - During prolonged plantar flexion, popliteal stenosis is detected

Conventional Angiography Findings
- Similar findings described above for MRA

Duplex Ultrasound Findings
- Similar findings to cross-sectional imaging; requires skilled sonographer

Imaging Recommendations
- MRI followed by contrast-enhanced MR angiography in neutral, plantar flexion, and dorsal flexion positions

Differential Diagnosis
Cystic Adventitial Disease (CAD)
- Rare condition, mucin collects in the adventitial layer of popliteal artery
- Relatively sudden onset calf pain and claudication
- MRA/angiographic appearance is of smooth, eccentric, extrinsic "hour-glass" narrowing of the popliteal artery in neutral position

Popliteal Entrapment

Popliteal Artery Aneurysm
- Patients with history of atherosclerotic and/or aneurysmal disease
- MRA/CTA/angiography demonstrates ectasia of popliteal artery

Popliteal Artery Embolism
- Abrupt onset of claudication
- Patient with history of embolic source
- Angiographic findings (MRA/CTA/angiography) demonstrate abrupt "cutoff" of popliteal artery with meniscus associated with embolus, and few collaterals

Pathology
General
- Generally regarded as congenital condition
- Etiology-Pathogenesis (see classification criteria for mechanism)
- Epidemiology
  - Male >> female, 15:1
  - Age 12-65 years, most less than 30 years
  - Incidence unknown, estimated at 0.165% of 20,000 Greek army patients
  - Bilateral in 22-67%

Microscopic Features
- Exam of the arterial segment demonstrates abundant longitudinal muscle fibers in the tunica media
- Internal elastic lamina is disrupted with fibrous thickening of intima

Staging or Grading Criteria
- Type I anomaly: Popliteal artery (PA) deviates medially around the medial head of the gastrocnemius muscle that arises close to its normal location
- Type II: Medial head of gastrocnemius muscle arises more laterally on femoral condyle
- Type III: PA is trapped by lateral slip of the medial gastrocnemius muscle
- Type IV: Popliteus muscle or deep fibrous band compresses PA

Clinical Issues
Presentation
- Athletic male complaining of claudication symptoms in absence of atherosclerosis, and absence of risk factors for atherosclerosis
- Not unusual for onset of symptoms to be sudden
- May complain of nocturnal cramps, numbness, paresthesias
- Acute thrombosis and/or distal embolization may occur if popliteal artery shows extensive post-stenotic dilatation and aneurysm formation

Treatment
- Transection of muscle or fibrous band with mobilization of popliteal artery
- Condition of popliteal artery dictates need for vascular intervention

Prognosis
- Excellent

Selected References
1. Forester BB et al: Comparison of two-dimensional time-of-flight dynamic magnetic resonance angiography with digital subtraction angiography in popliteal artery entrapment syndrome. Can Assoc Radiol J 48: 11, 1997
2. Hoelting T et al: Entrapment of the popliteal artery and its surgical management in a 20-year period. Br J Surg 84: 338, 1997
3. Collins PS et al: Popliteal artery entrapment: An evolving syndrome. J Vasc Surg 10: 484,1989

Femoropopliteal Artery Disease

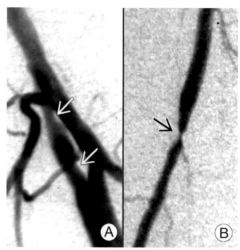

DSA images of SFA stenoses. (A) Two stenoses (arrows) of about 50% diameter-reduction are present just distal to the SFA origin. (B) Farther distal (mid thigh) a high-grade stenosis is present (arrow), measured at 70% diameter-reduction.

Key Facts
- Definition: Stenosis or occlusion of the common femoral artery (CFA), superficial femoral artery (SFA), or popliteal artery
- Classic imaging appearance
  - Arterial stenoses, common at CFA bifurcation, region of adductor canal or in popliteal artery
  - Collateral flow-implies chronicity, rather than acute obstruction
  - Post-stenotic dilatation distal to severe, chronic stenoses
  - Occlusion: Severe stenosis may progress to occlusion; thrombus forms above lesion and may propagate proximally

Imaging Findings
Ultrasound Findings
- Visible lumen narrowing on color Doppler, with post-stenotic turbulence
- Hemodynamically significant stenosis
  - Peak systolic velocity in stenosis = 2x velocity proximal to stenosis
  - Monophasic waveforms in stenosis
  - Damped waveforms distal to stenosis with high-grade obstruction
- Duplex ultrasound assessment is time intensive with limited use
CTA/MRA Findings
- High resolution femoropopliteal images possible with CTA and contrast-enhanced MRA; these methods rival contrast angiography accuracy but are not universally available
- Time-of-flight MRA technique inaccurate due to flow-related artifacts – contrast-enhanced MRA required
- Heavily calcified plaque limits usefulness of rendered images with CTA - need to include source images in interpretation
- CTA requires multidetector scanner, high contrast dose, rapid bolus injection, and sophisticated post-processing (risk of contrast reaction/ renal failure)

Femoropopliteal Artery Disease

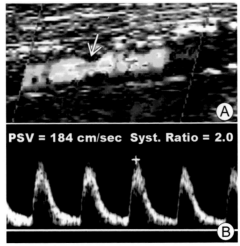

Color Doppler US of CFA stent stenosis. (A) The echogenic stent is easily seen. A focal stenosis is visible (arrow). (B) Peak systolic velocity (PSV) is 184 cm/sec and systolic velocity ratio 2.0. These values represent about 50% diameter reductions.

Angiography Findings
- See classic imaging appearance, above
- Angiography is current gold standard for characterization of arterial disease
- Minimally invasive, low risk (vessel injury, pseudoaneurysm)

Protocol for Assessment of Lower Extremity Arterial Insufficiency
- History and detailed physical examination focused on vascular system
- Ankle/brachial index, possibly segmental pressure or treadmill test
- If strong clinical evidence of localized inflow (iliac artery) disease
  - Limited imaging assessment may be satisfactory
  - Use CTA or MRA to confirm localized iliac disease
  - Proceed to percutaneous intervention or surgery
- If extent of disease is uncertain, based on clinical findings, or if there is evidence of femoropopliteal disease, or severe multilevel disease
  - Comprehensive assessment of lower extremity arteries required
  - CTA/MRA if appropriate equipment and expertise is available, or
  - Catheter angiography (gold standard)

Differential Diagnosis

Atherosclerosis
- Irregular or eccentric narrowing, especially at bifurcation of CFA, popliteal artery or tibioperitoneal trunk
- Extensive collateralization

Embolic Disease
- Smooth abrupt occlusion, usually at bifurcations
- Lack of collateral vessels
- Search for etiology: Proximal aneurysm, cardiac vegetations, atrial thrombus

Traumatic Occlusion
- Common cause in young

Femoropopliteal Artery Disease

  o Extremity fracture, penetrating injury

Vasculitis
- Uncommon in femoral and popliteal arteries (e.g., FMD)
- Typically affects tibial and peroneal arteries and foot arteries (e.g., Buerger's disease, Raynaud's disease)

Pathology
General
- Younger patients: Vasculitis, trauma more likely
- Older patients: Atherosclerosis more likely
- Etiology-Pathogenesis
  o Atherosclerotic intimal plaques
    ▪ From smooth muscle proliferation, extracellular lipid/collagen deposition, and inflammation
    ▪ Plaque projects into the vessel lumen, causing stenosis/occlusion
- Epidemiology (atherosclerotic obstruction)
  o Males >> Females
  o Incidence increases with age: 3% age 45-54 yrs, 6% age 55-64 yrs

Clinical Issues
Presentation
- Embolic occlusion - abrupt onset arterial insufficiency symptoms
- Atherosclerosis – gradual evolution of symptoms most common
- Intermittent claudication
  o Definition: Exercise-related pain (or other symptoms) worsening with activity, and subsiding after several minutes rest
  o Graded by distance patient is able to walk
  o Location of pain may indicate level of obstruction
    ▪ Thigh pain: External iliac, common femoral artery
    ▪ Calf pain: Femoropopliteal occlusive disease

Treatment
- Acute occlusive thrombus
  o Thrombolysis trial
  o Angioplasty occasionally successful
  o Surgical thrombectomy
- Atherosclerosis
  o Angioplasty/stent
    ▪ Temporizing measure, useful in selected patients
    ▪ Rapid re-stenosis
    ▪ Can delay graft surgery for 2 or 3 years
  o Surgical bypass
    ▪ Preferred for long-term durability
    ▪ Reversed vein bypass is standard
    ▪ Can revascularize to distal tibial and peroneal vessels, if needed

Selected References
1. Lenhart M et al: Contrast media-enhanced MR angiography of the lower extremity arteries using a dedicated peripheral vascular coil system. Rofo Fortschr Geb Rontgenstr Neuen Bildgeb Verfahr 172: 992-9, 2000
2. Rubin GD et al: Multi-detector row CT angiography of lower extremity arterial inflow and runoff: Initial experience. Radiology 221: 146-58, 2001
3. Kadir S: Teaching atlas of interventional radiology: Diagnostic and therapeutic angiography. Thieme, New York, 1999

Iliac Artery Disease

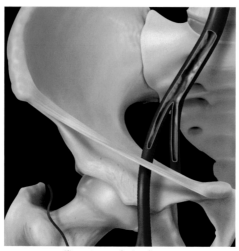

Iliac artery occlusive disease.

Key Facts
- Definition: Lower extremity inflow vessel stenosis or occlusion
- Classic imaging appearance
  - Arterial stenoses, usually at bifurcations
  - Collateral flow - implies chronicity, rather than acute obstruction
  - Post-stenotic dilatation distal to severe chronic stenoses
  - Occlusion
    - Severe stenosis may progress to occlusion
    - Thrombus forms above lesion and may propagate proximally

Imaging Findings
Duplex Ultrasound Findings
- Visible lumen narrowing on color Doppler, with post-stenotic turbulence
- Hemodynamically significant stenosis
  - Peak systolic velocity in stenosis = 2x velocity proximal to stenosis
  - Monophasic waveforms in stenosis
  - Damped waveforms distal to stenosis with high-grade obstruction
- Iliac artery duplex assessment often limited by obesity, bowel gas etc.
CTA/MRA Findings
- High resolution iliac images may be obtained with CTA and contrast-enhanced MRA, but these methods are not universally available
- Heavily calcified plaque may limit usefulness of rendered images, need to including source images in interpretation
- CTA requires multidetector scanner, high contrast dose, rapid bolus injection, and sophisticated post-processing (risk of contrast reaction and renal failure)
- Time-of-flight MRA technique inaccurate due to flow-related artifacts – contrast-enhanced MRA required
Angiography Findings
- Current gold standard for vessel characterization
- Minimally invasive, allows for percutaneous therapy

Iliac Artery Disease

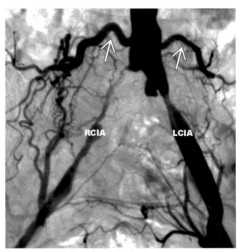

DSA, bilateral atherosclerotic iliac stenosis. A long segment, severe stenosis is present in the right common iliac artery (RCIA). A short segment, severe stenosis is present on the left (LCIA). Large lumbar collaterals (arrows) communicate with internal iliac artery branches.

- Minimally invasive

Protocol for Assessment of Lower Extremity Arterial Insufficiency
- History and detailed physical examination focused on vascular system
- Ankle/brachial index, possibly segmental pressure or treadmill test
- If strong clinical evidence of localized inflow (iliac artery) disease
  - Limited imaging assessment may be satisfactory
  - Use CTA or MRA to confirm localized iliac disease
  - Proceed to intervention or surgery (see treatment, below)
- If extent of disease is uncertain, based on clinical findings, or if there is evidence of multilevel arterial occlusive disease
  - Comprehensive assessment of lower extremity arteries required
  - CTA/MRA if appropriate equipment and expertise is available
  - Catheter angiography if CTA/MRA not available

Differential Diagnosis
Atherosclerosis
- Irregular or eccentric narrowing, especially at posterior aspect of aortic bifurcation, and in common iliac arteries
- Internal iliac stenosis common
- Extensive collateralization

Embolic Disease
- Acute or subacute symptoms
- Smooth abrupt occlusions, usually at bifurcations
- Lack of collateral vessels
- Search for etiology: Proximal aneurysm, cardiac vegetations, atrial thrombus

Traumatic Occlusion
- Most common cause of iliac occlusion in young
- Pelvic trauma

Iliac Artery Disease

- Catheterization-related injury (dissection, hematoma)

Pathology
General
- General Path Comments
  - Younger patients; vasculitis, tumor encasement, dissection more likely
  - Older patients: Atherosclerosis more likely
- Etiology-Pathogenesis
  - Atherosclerotic intimal plaques
    - From smooth muscle proliferation, extracellular lipid/collagen deposition, and inflammation
    - Plaque projects into the vessel lumen, causing stenosis/occlusion
- Epidemiology (atherosclerotic obstruction)
  - Males >> Females
  - Incidence increases with age: 3% age 45-54 yrs, 6% age 55-64 yrs

Clinical Issues
Presentation
- Intermittent claudication
  - Definition: Exercise-related pain (or other symptoms) worsening with activity, and subsiding after several minutes' rest
  - Graded by distance patient is able to walk
  - Location of pain may indicate level of obstruction
    - Buttock: Aorta, common iliac artery
    - Thigh: External iliac, common femoral artery
- Impotence
  - Diminished flow, internal iliac-, pudendal- and obturator arteries
- Leriche syndrome
  - Bilateral leg claudication, absence of femoral pulses, impotence
  - Cause: Aortic or bilateral common iliac artery obstruction
Treatment
- Acute occlusive thrombus
  - Thrombolysis trial
  - Angioplasty occasionally successful
  - Surgical thrombectomy
- Iliac stenosis
  - Focal (< 5 cm length)
    - Angioplasty with stent: 97% primary patency, 80-90% 5-year patency
  - Focal (> 5 cm length)
    - Surgical bypass or endarterectomy (gold standard for patency)
- Iliac occlusion, multifocal iliac disease, or aortic stenosis/occlusion
  - aortofemoral or axillofemoral graft
  - Percutaneous therapy can be tried but generally less effective

Selected References
1. Lenhart M et al: Contrast media-enhanced MR angiography of the lower extremity arteries using a dedicated peripheral vascular coil system. Rofo Fortschr Geb Rontgenstr Neuen Bildgeb Verfahr 172: 992-9, 2000
2. Rubin GD et al: Multi-detector row CT angiography of lower extremity arterial inflow and runoff: Initial experience. Radiology 221: 146-58, 2001
3. Kadir S: Teaching atlas of interventional radiology: Diagnostic and therapeutic angiography. Thieme, New York, 1999

Venous Thrombosis, Acute/Subacute

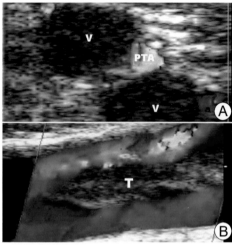

Acute venous thrombosis. (A) Short axis US image shows that the posterior tibial veins (V) do not collapse with compression. Note: flow absent, veins distended, thrombus hypoechoic and homogeneous. PTA = posterior tibial artery. (B) Long axis US image of free-floating thrombus (T) in the common femoral vein.

Key Facts
- Definition: Thrombosis of extremity veins
  - **Thrombophlebitis**: Acute, with adjacent tissue inflammation
  - **Subacute thrombosis**: Clot persists, but soft-tissue inflammation diminished or resolved (> 7-14 days)
- Risk of pulmonary embolization in acute phase

Imaging Findings
General Features
- Best imaging clue
  - Failure of veins to collapse during compresssion with US transducer
  - Occlusive or non-occlusive thrombus in vein lumen on US
CTV/MRV Findings
- Acute
  - Thrombus = filling defect in lumen, no signal MRV, low density CTV
  - Contrast flow around thrombus = "tram-track" appearance
  - Collateral veins (adjacent to thrombosed vein or distant)
  - Peri-venous inflammation
- Subacute
  - Thrombus retracts, vein is less distended
  - High T1 signal in thrombus due to T1 shortening from paramagnetic effect of methemoglobin
  - Variable lysis of thrombus and vein recanalization
Ultrasound Findings
- Lack of vein collapse with compression best sign of thrombus
- Acute
  - Vein markedly distended
  - Thrombus hypoechoic, homogeneous
  - Small flow streams around ("tram-track") and through thrombus
  - Free-floating thrombus (unattached proximal end)

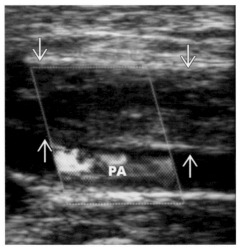

Subacute venous thrombus. Long axis view of three week old popliteal vein thrombus (arrows). Vein remains distended, compared with the popliteal artery (PA). Thrombus is more echogenic and heterogeneous than acute thrombus

- Subacute
  - Increased thrombus echogenicity/heterogeneity
  - Shrinkage of thrombus = decreased vein size
  - Variable restoration of flow
  - Collateralization

Venographic Findings
- Non-visualization of vein(s) (equivocal: Acute, chronic, or technical)
- Filling defect in vein lumen (equivocal: Acute or subacute)
- "Tram-track:" Classic acute, contrast flow around thrombus

Imaging Recommendations
- US is primary diagnostic method for extremity venous thrombosis
- Contrast venography if US technically flawed
- Pulmonary CTA or scintigraphy for pulmonary embolization (PE)
- CTV of femoropopliteal area after pulmonary CTA
- Overall, CTV and MRV not widely used, less accurate than US

Differential Diagnosis

Venous Congestion due to Central Vein Obstruction or CHF
- Obstruction = continuous Doppler flow (absence of respiratory variation)
- CHF = pulsatile Doppler flow in lower extremity veins

Lymphatic Obstruction

Ruptured Popliteal Cyst

Muscle Tear, Soft-Tissue Hematoma

Pathology

General
- Thrombosis often precipitated by a combination of factors
- Endothelial cells have role in thrombus formation (poorly understood)
- Inflammation of vein wall follows thrombus formation: Thrombophlebitis = thrombosis + phlebitis (vein wall inflammation)

Venous Thrombosis, Acute/Subacute

- Thrombus stages and evolution
  - Acute: Fresh coagulum, poorly attached to vein wall, inflammation
  - Subacute: Resolution of inflammation, thrombus retraction and adherence to wall, variable lysis
  - Chronic
- Pathogenesis
  - Endothelial damage (e.g., indwelling line, infection, caustic infusion)
  - Venous stasis (e.g., immobility, neoplastic vein compression, pregnancy)
  - Hypercoagulable states
    - Intrinsic hematologic disorder
    - Neoplasia-induced hypercoagulability (migratory thrombophlebitis): Increased factor VIII causes enhanced thromboplastin production
    - Hemoconcentration (e.g., erythroid leukemia, dehydration)
- Genetics
  - Recurrent thrombosis from several clotting factor abnormalities

Clinical Issues
Superficial vs. Deep Vein Thrombosis (DVT)
- Superficial thrombophlebitis = uncommon source of PE and venous insufficiency, usually not treated with anticoagulation
- DVT = common source of PE (especially iliac, femoral, popliteal, subclavian and axillary veins), anticoagulation routine

Presentation/Diagnosis
- 40-50% of lower extremity DVT cases asymptomatic
- Extremity swelling
- Pain, varying from dull ache to severe discomfort, diffuse or localized
- Focal tenderness to palpation, from inflammation (especially calf)
- Palpable tender "cord" (acutely thrombosed superficial vein)
- Phlegmasia alba, or cerulea, dolens: Swollen, painful, blanched (alba) or cyanotic (cerulea) extremity, from extensive acute venous thrombosis
- Dyspnea, hypoxemia, chest pain, from acute PE
- **Negative extremity vein examination does not exclude PE**

Natural History
- Acute thrombophlebitis gives way to subacute thrombosis in 7-14 days
- Variable degree of thrombus lysis in subacute period (weeks/months)
- Residual thrombus becomes scar

Treatment & Prognosis
- Anticoagulation, initially with heparin then with warfarin (usually 3 months)
- Thrombolysis should be considered especially in young patients with severe ileofemoral thrombosis
- IVC filter placement if patient has contradiction to or failure of complication of anticoagulation
- Related to the extent and cause of thrombosis, degree of lysis vs. organization, and resultant severity of venous insufficiency

Selected References
1. Peterson DA et al: Computed tomographic venography is specific but not sensitive for diagnosis of acute lower-extremity deep venous thrombosis in patients with suspected pulmonary embolus. J Vasc Surg 34: 798-804, 2001
2. Browse NL et al: Diseases of the Veins, Ed2: London, Arnold, 249-317, 1999
3. Cronan JJ: Venous thromboembolic disease: the role of US. Radiology 186: 619-30, 1993

Venous Thrombosis, Chronic

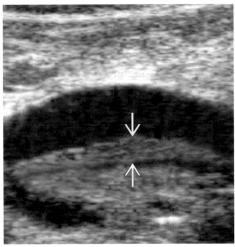

Post-thrombotic scar. Long axis view of a popliteal vein shows fibrotic thickening (arrows) of the vein wall 18 months post acute thrombosis.

Key Facts
- Definition: Chronic sequelae of extremity venous thrombosis
- Thrombus that does not lyse becomes fibrous tissue (scar)
- Possible debilitating venous stasis

Imaging Findings
General Features
- Best imaging clues
  - Vein wall thickening
  - Reduced vein caliber
  - Occlusion
  - Collaterals persisting long after acute episode

CTV, MRV Findings
- Focal or diffuse vein wall thickening
- Synechiae (webs) or focal filling defects (the latter may be mistaken for acute/subacute thrombus)
- Reduced vein lumen caliber or occlusion
- Collaterals, along affected vein or at distant locations

Ultrasound (US) Findings
- Same as CTV/MRV, plus
  - Stiff, non-compressible veins
  - Focal plaque-like thickening of vein wall
  - Venous reflux (reversed flow) due to valvular incompetence
  - Incompetent perforator veins
- US assessment of venous incompetence (reflux)
  - Tailor examination to surgeon's needs (talk with surgeon)
  - Examine both superficial and deep veins
  - Determine what veins are normal, stenotic, occluded, varicose
  - Assess all areas for reflux (retrograde flow) and grade severity
  - Search for incompetent perforator veins (especially with skin ulceration)

Venous Thrombosis, Chronic

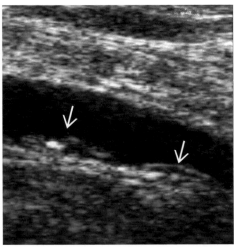

Plaque-like scars (arrows) are seen in a superficial femoral vein 2 years post acute thrombosis.

<u>Venographic Findings</u>
- Same as CTV/MRV, plus
  - Non-visualization of vein(s) due to occlusion
  - Irregular, tortuous, small caliber veins
  - Synechiae or filling defects in vein lumen

<u>Imaging Recommendations</u>
- US is primary diagnostic method for chronic extremity venous thrombosis and venous incompetence (reflux)
- Contrast venography if US technically flawed
- CTV and MRV not widely used for chronic venous disease

Differential Diagnosis
<u>Venous Congestion, Central Vein Obstruction or CHF (No Thrombosis), Lymphatic Obstruction</u>

Pathology
<u>General</u>
- Anticoagulation (heparin, warfarin) prevents propagation of existing thrombus but does not lyse thrombus
- Intrinsic mechanisms of thrombolysis
  - Vein epithelial cells, and other cells, produce plasminogen activators which activate circulating plasminogen, forming plasmin
  - Plasmin (an enzyme) breaks down clot fibrin into soluble products
- Therapeutic mechanisms of thrombolysis
  - Plasminogen activators administered systemically or directly into thrombus via catheter
  - Due to concern for hemorrhage, therapeutic thrombolysis is used uncommonly for extremity venous thrombosis, should probably be used more often especially in young patients with acute thrombosis of ileofemoral vein
- Possible modes of venous thrombus evolution

Venous Thrombosis, Chronic

- o Rapid lysis of thrombus, with little or no residual clot
- o Focal areas of residual, un-lysed thrombus
- o Extensive residual, un-lysed thrombus
- o Note: Incomplete lysis is **very common** (up to 80% of lower extremity DVT cases)
- Un-lysed thrombus adheres to vein wall, is invaded by fibroblasts, forming fibrous tissue (scar), which evolves over many months
- Potential outcomes of venous scar formation
  - o Vein becomes a fibrotic cord (occluded, small caliber)
  - o Circumferential vein wall thickening, with reduced caliber, but patent
    - Focal stenosis
    - Diffusely narrowed
  - o Focal vein wall thickening (non-circumferential), with wide patency
  - o Synechiae (fibrous tissue webs) or focal fibrous tissue masses (filling defects), with wide patency
- Thrombosis damages vein valves
  - o Thrombosis alone, without scar formation, **may** damage valves
  - o All valves **certainly** damaged in areas of scar formation
  - o Potential extent of valve damage depends on extent of thrombosis
  - o Damaged valves are incompetent, allowing retrograde blood flow and causing venous stasis
  - o Stasis-induced venous pressure elevation interferes with capillary drainage, leading to soft-tissue edema
  - o Chronic edema and stasis cause tissue hypoxemia, skin ulceration, and secondary incompetence of perforator veins (from dilatation)

Clinical Issues

Chronic Venous Stasis
- Synonyms: Post-thrombotic limb syndrome, chronic venous insufficiency
- Common: Follows 50-60% of lower extremity DVT episodes
- Very debilitating: Chronic edema, pain, possible skin ulceration

Calf Vein Thrombosis, a Therapeutic Dilemma
- Pulmonary embolization risk low from calf, anticoagulation not required
- Does anticoagulation prevent/ameliorate chronic venous stasis
  - o Evidence to date not convincing
  - o Studies are inadequate

Prognosis
- Surgery for post-thrombotic venous stasis has limited success
- Post-thrombotic venous stasis cannot be cured, can be ameliorated by conservative measures (e.g., limb elevation, compressive stockings)

Selected References
1. Browse NL et al: Diseases of the Veins, Ed2: London, Arnold, 319-58 and 386-408, 1999
2. Lynch TG et al: Developments in diagnosis and classification of venous disorders: Non-invasive diagnosis. Cardiovasc Surg 7: 160-78, 1999
3. Weingarten MS: Distribution and quantification of venous reflux in lower extremity chronic venous stasis disease with duplex scanning. J Vasc Surg 18: 753-9, 1993

Venous Insufficiency

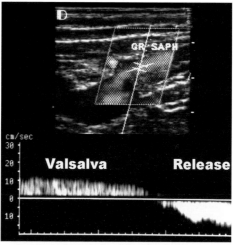

Venous reflux. Sustained retrograde flow (above baseline) is present in the greater saphenous vein during the Valsalva maneuver. The normal flow direction resumes with Valsalva release. Normally, flow should cease during Valsalva.

Key Facts
- Synonyms: Venous reflux, venous incompetence, venous stasis
- Definition: Disordered function of lower extremity veins resulting from valvular insufficiency
- Classic imaging appearance
  - Retrograde flow in lower extremity veins with Valsalva maneuver
- Other key facts
  - Results in chronic venous stasis, chronic edema, and soft-tissue injury
  - Major cause of disability

Imaging Findings
Best Imaging Clue
- Sustained flow reversal in lower extremity veins on color- or spectral Doppler ultrasound (US) examination
Normal Venous Ultrasound Findings
- Veins patent, no evidence of chronic scarring (see "Chronic Thrombosis")
- Spontaneous cephalad blood flow in large extremity veins
- Abrupt ($\leq$ 0.5 second) cessation of venous flow with the Valsalva maneuver, or manual compression proximal to examination site
- Blood flow in perforating calf veins only from superficial to deep system; perforating vein diameter 3 mm or less
Abnormal Venous Ultrasound Findings
- Sustained venous flow reversal (venous reflux) with the Valsalva maneuver or compression proximal to the examination site
- Reflux grades
  - Various grading systems in different medical institutions; some simply note presence or absence of reflux
  - < 3 sec. popliteal vein (v.) reflux correlates with mild clinical symptoms (edema, venous congestion, varicosities)

Venous Insufficiency

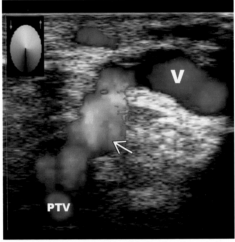

Incompetent perforating vein. A massively dilated perforating vein (arrow) connects a posterior tibial vein (PTV) with a superficial varicose vein (V). Orange color indicates reflux from the deep system (PTV) to the superficial system.

- o > 3 sec popliteal vein reflux correlates with more severe symptoms including skin changes and ulceration
- o Salt Lake City VA Medical center grading criteria
  - ▪ Reflux ≤ 2 sec, Grade 1
  - ▪ Reflux 2-3 sec, Grade 2
  - ▪ Reflux > 3 sec, Grade 3
- Dilated, incompetent perforating veins
  - o Diameter > 3 mm
  - o Flow from deep to superficial system
- Other vein abnormalities
  - o Venous occlusion, chronic scarring, collateralization
  - o Vein dilatation (does not correlate well with clinical abnormality)
  - o Varicosities (usually superficial veins)

Examination Protocol for Lower Extremity Venous Dysfunction
- Patient 45° reverse Trendelenburg
- Examine deep and superficial veins for patency and normality, note areas of occlusion, scar, collateralization
- Obtain common femoral v. Doppler signals (rule out proximal obstruction)
- Use color Doppler to test for reflux, with Valsalva maneuver, in superficial femoral v., popliteal v., posterior tibial v's, peroneal v's, greater saphenous v. (mid thigh and below knee) and lesser saphenous v.
- In areas where color Doppler shows reflux, grade with spectral Doppler
- Skin thickening and ulceration: Search for incompetent perforating veins
- Surgical planning: Know what information surgeon needs before you start examination

Imaging Recommendations
- Color Doppler US is the primary modality for assessing lower extremity venous dysfunction; other modalities have largely been abandoned
- A new air plethysmography method has been proposed for classifying reflux severity

Venous Insufficiency

- Venography particular to evaluate iliac veins

Differential Diagnosis
Lymphedema
- Normal venous system without venous reflux
Venous Congestion (e.g., CHF, Venous Compression or Occlusion in Abdomen)
- Veins distended but patent, no reflux, continuous flow in CFV
- On left consider May-Thurner syndrome

Pathology
General
- Anatomy/Physiology
  - Venous valves are bicuspid
  - Valves increasingly numerous from the thigh to foot (1-2 cm apart in calf)
  - Blood is propelled forward in veins solely by muscular compression
- Etiology-Pathogenesis (chronic venous stasis)
  - Thrombosis-induced scarring destroys valves, obstructs flow by occlusion or stenosis – primary cause of chronic venous insufficiency
  - Protein-rich soft-tissue edema causes metabolic changes / inflammation
  - Calf skin becomes "woody" (lipodermatosclerosis) and may ulcerate
  - Diapedesis of red cells, and cell breakdown causes brown skin color
- Etiology (superficial varicose veins)
  - Greater or lesser saphenous incompetence (primary or post-thrombotic)
  - Deep venous system occlusion, with collateral flow to superficial system
  - Incompetent perforating veins in calf

Clinical Issues
Presentation
- Various levels of disability
  - Varicose veins (primarily a cosmetic issue)
  - Mild extremity edema and "heavy" feeling
  - Severe extremity swelling, skin changes, ulceration, and severe debility
Treatment
- Supportive measures, surgery for specific problems
- Percutaneous laser ablation is therapy for greater sapheous reflux
- Sclerotherapy possible for smaller superficial vaciosoties
Prognosis
- Good for varicosities and mild stasis symptoms
- Poor for severe chronic insufficiency

Selected References
1. Bundens WP et al: Definitive diagnosis and documentation of chronic venous dysfunction. [In] Zwiebel WJ: Introduction to vascular ultrasonography. Philadelphia, WB Saunders, 347-68, 2000
2. Lynch TG et al: Developments in diagnosis and classification of venous disorders: Non-invasive diagnosis. Cardiovasc Surg 7: 160-78, 1999
3. Weingarten MS et al: Distribution and quantification of venous reflux in lower extremity chronic venous stasis disease with duplex scanning. J Vasc Surg 18: 753-9, 1993

Buerger's Disease

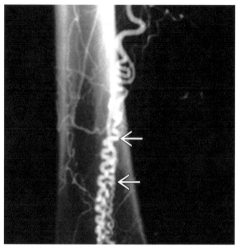

"Corkscrew" collaterals (arrows) are characteristic of Buerger's disease. Although found with Buerger's disease, they are not pathognomonic for Buerger's and are seen in other vascular diseases where occlusions or long segment stenoses occur.

Key Facts
- Synonym: Thromboangiitis obliterans
- Definition: Inflammatory disease affecting arteries and veins causing stenoses and occlusions of the vessels
- Classic imaging appearance: Stenoses and occlusions of multiple medium to small vessels, calf arteries and forearm arteries are commonly involved
- Occurs in heavy smokers, tobacco is the sole known etiologic factor
- Bilateral leg claudication in a young, heavy smoker is classic

Imaging Findings
General Features
- Best imaging clue: Angiogram demonstrating small vessels of calf and foot with bilateral multifocal segmental occlusions or severe stenoses
- "Corkscrew" collaterals

CT Findings
- Not commonly performed, if CECT scan with 3D reconstruction was performed, findings would be those seen with angiography

MR Findings
- Not commonly performed, 2D time-of-flight could be performed and the findings would be those seen with angiography

Ultrasound Findings
- Not commonly performed; since veins can be involved, if an ultrasound was performed in a patient with phlebitis, thickening of the vein and/or artery walls might be observed, also multiple collaterals might be noted

Angiography Findings
- Small vessels of calf and foot, or forearm and hand, are affected
- Lower extremity involvement
  - Anterior tibial, posterior tibial, peroneal arteries, plantar arteries; popliteal artery less frequently involved
  - Vessels proximal to popliteal are almost always normal

Buerger's Disease

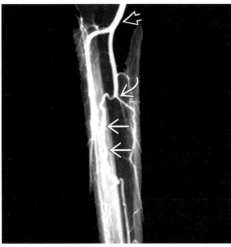

Buerger's disease is characterized by proximal arteries which are normal in appearance (open arrow) and then abrupt occlusions (curved arrow) with very tortuous collaterals (arrows).

- Upper extremity
  - Radial, ulnar interosseus arteries, palmar and digital arteries are involved
  - Rarely brachial artery or proximal upper extremity artery involvement
- Bilateral, focal or multifocal, segmental occlusions
- Abrupt transitions from normal caliber vessel to diseased or occluded vessel
- Lumen above the thrombosed segments is smooth and narrow without evidence of arterial wall irregularity
- Extensive, tortuous collateral system is present
- "Corkscrew" or "corrugated" collaterals – not pathognomonic for Buerger's and have been seen in other diseases with diffuse arterial narrowing and occlusions

Imaging Recommendations
- Angiography should be the diagnostic procedure of choice, although MRA could be performed with compromised renal function (rare)

Differential Diagnosis

Atherosclerosis
- Although uncommon, accelerated atherosclerosis may be seen in young patients
- More commonly the large and medium-sized arteries involvement
- Although patients may be young for atherosclerotic disease, if they started smoking as pre-teen, they may have a significant pack-year smoking history

Vasculitis
- More common in upper extremity
- Small and medium-sized arteries
- Associated with multiple collagen vascular disorders
- Often associated with Raynaud's phenomena

Buerger's Disease

Pathology
General
- Both arteries and veins may be involved
- Etiology-Pathogenesis
  - Tobacco use is the sole known etiological factor and is thought to trigger the disease through an autoimmune mechanism
- Epidemiology
  - Young adult males – heavy smoker
  - Disease rarely occurs in women (less than 2%), although the incidence appears to be increasing probably because of the increasing number of women smokers

Microscopic Features
- Non-necrotizing panarteritis involving medium and small arteries of the extremities
- Walls of arteries or veins or both are swollen with a moderate cellular infiltrate of the adventitia and media
- Lumen occluded by highly cellular thrombus containing characteristic microabscesses

Clinical Issues
Presentation
- Bilateral claudication
- Pedal pulses may be present, but usually they are diminished or absent
- Rest pain, ulceration and gangrene may be present
- Superficial migratory phlebitis

Natural History
- If patients continue smoking, it is common for disease to progress to amputation

Treatment
- Very difficult to treat
- Angioplasty very difficult in these very small arteries with multifocal disease
- Surgery very difficult to bypass because all of the distal target sites for by pass are diseased, vein grafts may not be possible if the veins are involved with the process

Prognosis
- Poor, unless patients stop smoking
- These patients find it extraordinarily difficult to stop smoking

Selected References
1. Diehm C et al: Thromboangiitis obliterans (Buerger's disease). NEJM 344: 230-1, 2001
2. Nakajima N: The change in concept and surgical treatment on Buerger's disease-personal experience and review. Int J Cardiol 66: S273-80, 1998
3. Olin JW: Thromboangiitis obliterans (Buerger's disease). NEJM 343: 864-69, 2000

Musculoskeletal Angiomatosis

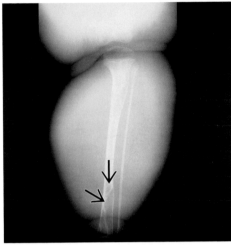

Congenital lymphangiomatosis of the leg in a 6-year-old boy. Note mixed lytic-sclerotic bone destruction (arrows). (Courtesy Drs Murphey and Kransdorf)

Key Facts
- Synonym: Combined hemangiomatosis and lymphangiomatosis
- Definition: Extensive angiomatous infiltration of one or more tissues; e.g., bone (most common), skin, muscle, viscera, subcutaneous fat
- Classic imaging appearance: Infiltrating, enhancing soft tissue mass
- Usually found in children and young adults
- May be associated with syndromes
  - Maffucci's: Multiple enchondromas and soft-tissue hemangiomas
  - Osler-Weber-Rendu: Fibromuscular dysplasia of all vessels resulting in telangiectasias, angiomas, and AVMs with bleeding
  - Klippel-Trenaunay-Weber: Triad of cutaneous hemangiomas, varicose veins, and soft tissue hypertrophy
  - Kasabach-Merritt: Thrombocytopenia resulting from intravascular coagulation within angiomatous lesions
  - Gorham's Disease: Aka "disappearing bone disease," massive osteolysis from proliferating endothelial-lined vascular channels

Imaging Findings
General Features
- Best imaging clue
  - If primarily hemangioma: Osteolysis on plain film with associated soft-tissue mass and phleboliths
  - If primarily lymphangioma: Cystic or cavernous soft tissue mass of neck or axilla
CT Findings (Hemangioma Component)
- NECT: Lytic ("lattice work") destruction of bone with soft tissue mass and phleboliths
- CECT: Same as above except mass enhances
CT Findings (Lymphangioma Component)
- Soft-tissue mass of neck or axilla in infant with septations which may enhance (but no vascular channels)

Musculoskeletal Angiomatosis

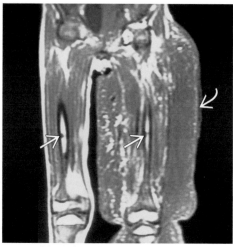

Lymphangiomatosis of the thigh in a 6-year-old boy. Note gigantism (curved arrow) and bilateral bony lesions (arrows) on this T1W coronal image (same patient as previous page). (Courtesy Drs Murphey and Kransdorf)

- Focal gigantism
- Lymphedema
- Cystic hygroma
- Thoracic involvement may cause chylothorax
- Abdominal involvement may cause chyloperitoneum, hepatosplenomegaly

MR Findings
- T1WI: Hypointense soft-tissue mass; hemangioma component contains central vascular channels and peripheral fat overgrowth
- T2WI: Hyperintense intramuscular or intraosseus soft tissue mass
- T1WI with contrast: Hemangioma - vascular channels enhance; lymphangioma - septations may enhance
- STIR or fat-saturated T2 FSE: Most sensitive for subtle disease

Ultrasound
- Multiloculated complex, cystic mass (lymphangioma component)

Imaging Recommendations
- MRI with STIR and T1WI with and without contrast

Differential Diagnosis

Hemangioma
- No lymphangiomatous component; less infiltrating

Lymphangioma
- Usually soft tissue only (neck and axilla); rarely involves bone

Spindle Cell Tumor (Benign or Malignant)
- Generally isointense to muscle on T2WI
- Soft-tissue mass lacks vascular channels (hemangiomatous component) and complex, cystic mass (lymphangiomatous component)

Pathology

General
- General Path Comments

Musculoskeletal Angiomatosis

- o Infiltrating combined hemangiomatous and lymphangiomatous soft tissue mass
- o Genetics (only with some syndromes)
  - Osler-Weber-Rendu (hereditary hemorrhagic telangiectasia)
  - Nonne-Milroy-Meige syndrome (congenital elephantiasis) is primarily lymphangiomatous and inherited in autosomal dominant pattern
- Etiology: Mixed causes
  - o Lymphangiomatous component due to obstructed lymphatic channels
  - o Gorham's disease: 50% have history of antecedent trauma

Gross Pathologic or Surgical Features
- Infiltrating hemangiomatous and lymphangiomatous soft tissue and osseous masses

Microscopic Features
- Dilated endothelial-lined vascular (hemangioma) or lymphatic (lymphangioma) channels infiltrating multiple tissues

Staging or Grading Criteria
- Based on size of channel, e.g., "cavernous," "cystic," etc.

Clinical Issues
Presentation
- Prominent, painful, bluish soft-tissue mass

Natural History
- Progressive infiltration despite attempted treatment

Treatment: Difficult Due to Tendency to Recur; Multiple Therapies Needed
- Surgical resection (90% recurrence despite "benign" classification)
- Embolotherapy
- Sclerotherapy
- Radiation

Prognosis
- Best with combined therapy
- Worst with lymphangiomatous visceral involvement
- Low malignant potential (except Maffucci's)
- Recurrences common

Selected References
1. Levey DS et al: Cystic angiomatosis: Case report and review of the literature. Skeletal Radiol 25: 287, 1996
2. Rao VK et al: Angiomatosis of soft tissue: An analysis of the histologic features and clinical outcome in 51 cases. Am J Surg Pathol 16: 764, 1992
3. Huvos AG: Hemangioma, lymphangioma, angiomatosis/lymphangiomatosis, glomus tumor. In Huvos AG, ed: Bone tumors: diagnosis, treatment and prognosis, ed 2, Philadelphia, W.B. Saunders, 1991

Musculoskeletal Hemangioendothelioma

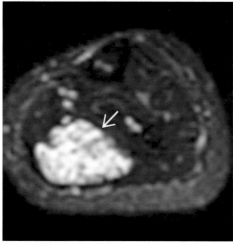

Axial STIR image of hemangioendothelioma of calf in 7-year-old boy (arrow).

Key Facts

- Definition: Tumor arising from vascular endothelial cells
- Benign or malignant
- Classic imaging appearance: Enhancing soft tissue or osseous tumor with peripheral vascular flow voids on MRI
- Soft tissue vs. osseous location depends on age and gender
  - Young patients: Tumor usually intramuscular, lower extremity
    - 50% arise next to a vessel
  - Young men (2nd – 3rd decade): Osseous lesions more common
    - Typically involve calvarium, spine, or long bones of lower extremity
  - In older adults (30-65), hemangiopericytoma more likely
    - Usually soft-tissue mass
  - In elderly patients with chronic lymphedema, consider angiosarcoma
    - Especially following mastectomy (Stewart-Treves syndrome)
    - Hemangioendothelioma cannot be distinguished radiographically from hemangiopericytoma or angiosarcoma

Imaging Findings

General Features
- Best imaging clue: Soft-tissue or osseous tumor with macroscopic vessels

CT Findings
- NECT: Nonspecific mass involving soft tissue or bone; aggressive tumors demonstrate bony erosion
- CECT: Enhancing mass involving soft tissue or bone

MR Findings
- T1WI: Soft-tissue or osseous tumor isointense to muscle
- T2WI: Hyperintense soft-tissue or osseous tumor
  - Gadolinium-enhanced T1WI: Enhancing tumor of soft tissue or bone

Other Modality Findings
- DSA: Aggressive tumors demonstrate
  - Dense vascular blush

Musculoskeletal Hemangioendothelioma

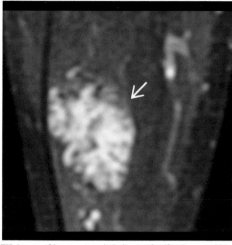

Sagittal STIR image of hemangioendothelioma of calf in 7-year-old boy (arrow).

  o Arteriovenous shunting
  o Early venous filling
<u>Imaging Recommendations</u>
- MRI with contrast demonstrates nonspecific enhancing mass of soft tissue or bone and vascular flow voids

Differential Diagnosis
<u>Hemangiopericytoma</u>
- Patients older than those with hemangioendothelioma, e.g., 30-65 yo
- Typically soft tissue mass of lower extremity or retroperitoneum
<u>Angiosarcoma</u>
- Patients much older than those with hemangioblastoma
- Often associated with chronic lymphedema
- May involve skin; could simulate Kaposi's sarcoma
<u>Less Common</u>
- Alveolar soft tissue sarcoma, alveolar rhabdomyosarcoma, synovial sarcoma, and extraskeletal Ewing's sarcoma

Pathology
<u>General</u>
- Nonspecific tumor arising from vascular endothelium
  o Hypervascular, often adjacent to blood vessel
  o Cannot be distinguished radiologically from hemangiopericytoma
- Genetics
  o Hemangioendothelioma may be associated with angiomatous syndromes
    ▪ Kasabach-Merritt
    ▪ Maffucci's
    ▪ Klippel-Trenaunay-Weber
    ▪ Congenital lymphedema
- Epidemiology

Musculoskeletal Hemangioendothelioma

- o Children: Deep, intramuscular tumor of lower extremity
- o Young men: Osseous tumor of bone (cranium, spine, leg)

Gross Pathologic or Surgical Features
- Hypervascular mass of soft tissue or bone
- Soft tissue lesions usually intramuscular lower extremity
- Bony lesions lytic and occasionally expansile
  - o Can occasionally break through cortex, leading to adjacent soft tissue mass

Microscopic Features
- Tumor arising from vascular endothelial cells; subtypes
  - o Epithelioid, spindle cell, and Kaposiform
- Benign or malignant
  - o Features of malignancy: Initial mass > 5 cm, high mitotic index, hemorrhage or necrosis, high cellularity, and immaturity

Clinical Issues
Presentation
- Nonspecific hypervascular mass which can be benign or malignant (low grade)
  - o Children: Intramuscular mass of leg
  - o Young men: Lytic bony mass of skull, spine, or legs

Treatment
- Surgical excision
- Adjuvant chemotherapy and radiation for more aggressive tumors

Prognosis
- Favorable with surgical resection
- 13% local recurrence; 31% metastasis (half of which are lethal)

Selected References
1. Murphey MD et al: Musculoskeletal angiomatous lesions. In magnetic resonance imaging (3rd Ed) Stark DD, Bradley WG (Eds), Mosby, St Louis, 1999
2. Enzinger FM et al: Hemangioendothelioma: Vascular tumors of intermediate malignancy. In Enzinger FM, and Weiss SW, eds: Soft tissue tumors, ed 3, Mosby, St Louis, 1995
3. Steinbach LS et al: MR imaging of spindle cell hemangioendothelioma. J Comput Assist Tomogr 15: 155, 1991

Index of Diagnoses

NOTES

NOTES

NOTES

_____
_____
_____
_____
_____
_____
_____
_____
_____
_____
_____
_____
_____
_____
_____
_____
_____
_____
_____
_____
_____
_____
_____
_____

NOTES

NOTES

NOTES

NOTES

NOTES

NOTES

NOTES

NOTES

NOTES

NOTES

NOTES